Nutritional Coaching Strategy to Modulate Training Efficiency

Nestlé Nutrition Institute Workshop Series

Vol. 75

Nutritional Coaching Strategy to Modulate Training Efficiency

Editors

Kevin D. Tipton Stirling, Scotland, UK
Luc J.C. van Loon Maastricht, The Netherlands

KARGER

Nestlé Nutrition Institute

Nestec Ltd., 55 Avenue Nestlé, CH–1800 Vevey (Switzerland)
S. Karger AG, P.O. Box, CH–4009 Basel (Switzerland) www.karger.com

Library of Congress Cataloging-in-Publication Data

Nutritional coaching strategy to modulate training efficiency / editors,
Kevin D. Tipton, Luc J.C. van Loon.
    p. ; cm. -- (Nestlé nutrition institute workshop series, ISSN
1664-2147 ; v. 75)
  Includes bibliographical references and index.
  ISBN 978-3-318-02332-9 (hardcover : alk. paper) -- ISBN 978-3-318-02333-6
(e-ISBN)
  I. Tipton, Kevin D. II. Loon, Luc J. C. van. III. Nestlé Nutrition
Institute. IV. Series: Nestlé Nutrition Institute workshop series ; v. 75.
1664-2147
  [DNLM: 1. Nutritional Physiological Phenomena. 2. Dietary Supplements.
3. Exercise Tolerance--physiology. 4. Physical Fitness--physiology. W1
NE228D / QU 145]
  RM216
  615.8'54--dc23
                                                    2013002890

The material contained in this volume was submitted as previously unpublished material, except in the instances in which credit has been given to the source from which some of the illustrative material was derived.
  Great care has been taken to maintain the accuracy of the information contained in the volume. However, neither Nestec Ltd. nor S. Karger AG can be held responsible for errors or for any consequences arising from the use of the information contained herein.
© 2013 Nestec Ltd., Vevey (Switzerland) and S. Karger AG, Basel (Switzerland). All rights reserved. This book is protected by copyright. No part of it may be reproduced, stored in a retrieval system, or transmitted, in any form or by any means, electronic, mechanical, photocopying, or recording, or otherwise, without the written permission of the publisher.

Printed on acid-free and non-aging paper (ISO 9706)
ISBN 978–3–318–02332–9
e-ISBN 978–3–318–02333–6
ISSN 1664–2147
e-ISSN 1664–2155

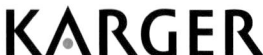 Basel · Freiburg · Paris · London · New York · New Delhi · Bangkok ·
Beijing · Tokyo · Kuala Lumpur · Singapore · Sydney

Contents

VII **Preface**
IX **Foreword**
XIII **Contributors**

1 **Nutritional Strategies to Modulate the Adaptive Response to Endurance Training**
Hawley, J.A. (Australia)

15 **Practical Considerations for Bicarbonate Loading and Sports Performance**
Burke, L.M. (Australia)

27 **Influence of Dietary Nitrate Supplementation on Exercise Tolerance and Performance**
Jones, A.M.; Vanhatalo, A.; Bailey, S.J. (UK)

41 **Nutritional Strategies to Support Adaptation to High-Intensity Interval Training in Team Sports**
Gibala, M.J. (Canada)

51 **Dietary Strategies to Attenuate Muscle Loss during Recovery from Injury**
Tipton, K.D. (UK)

63 **The New Carbohydrate Intake Recommendations**
Jeukendrup, A. (UK)

73 **Role of Dietary Protein in Post-Exercise Muscle Reconditioning**
van Loon, L.J.C. (The Netherlands)

85 **Nutritional Support to Maintain Proper Immune Status during Intense Training**
Gleeson, M. (UK)

99 **Use of β-Alanine as an Ergogenic Aid**
Derave, W. (Belgium)

109 **Vitamin D Supplementation in Athletes**
Larson-Meyer, E. (USA)

123 **Weight Management in the Performance Athlete**
Manore, M.M. (USA)

135 **Concluding Remarks: Nutritional Strategies to Support the Adaptive Response to Prolonged Exercise Training**
van Loon, L.J.C. (The Netherlands); Tipton, K.D. (UK)

143 **Subject Index**

For more information on related publications, please consult the NNI website: www.nestlenutrition-institute.org

Preface

In addition to regular training, nutrition is one of the key factors that modulate exercise performance. A healthy diet, adapted to the specific demands imposed upon by the individual athlete's training and competition, is required to allow optimal performance.Despite the fact that most athletes are primarily preoccupied with diet and nutritional support prior to and during exercise competition, there is an increasing awareness that nutrition plays a key role in translating the many training hours into useful adaptive responses in various tissues. Research over the last decade has shown many examples of the impact of dietary intervention to modulate the skeletal muscle adaptive response to prolonged exercise training. Of course, the latter is not surprising as it is the adaptive response to each successive exercise bout that results in a training status that allows peak performance. Therefore, proper nutritional coaching should not be restricted to the competitive events, but needs to be applied throughout both training and competition, each with itsspecific requirements regarding nutrient provision.

Proper nutritional counseling will improve exercise training efficiency and ultimately increase performance capacity. The latter is obviously of relevance for the competitive athlete, but also has important health and clinical relevance. In many preventative and therapeutic strategies, exercise has become accepted as a cornerstone in disease management. However, severely deconditioned people and more clinically compromised patient groups generally suffer from exercise intolerance limiting the volume and intensity of the exercise that can be performed. In these conditions, a more efficient adaptive response to an increase in habitual physical activity and/or exercise training would likely translate to greater clinical benefits. Clearly, the relevance of dietary counseling to modulate training efficiency will not be restricted to the competitive athlete, but extends to the general public and the more frail clinically compromised patient groups.

The aim of this workshop was to explore the numerous properties of nutritional interventions to modulate the adaptive response to exercise training and, as such, to identify nutritional strategies that improve exercise training efficiency. We hope that the following chapters will provide a solid scientific basis upon which the reader canredefine key targets for future interventionsand develop new insights into the complex interaction between nutrition and exercise.

Kevin D. Tipton
Luc J.C. van Loon

Foreword

Over the last few decades, much of sports nutrition research has focused on how to improve performance on race day, and many athletes likewise pay more attention to their race day nutrition than they do during the relatively larger volume of time they dedicate to training. There is a growing body of evidence, however, relating to the role that nutrition can play in helping athletes during training to get more out of their accumulated efforts as they prepare for competition. The concept that these nutritional strategies could be worked into an overall coaching regimen to help athletes improve over time was the overarching theme for the 75th Nestlé Nutrition Institute Workshop held in Majorca, Spain on the 7–8th of December 2011.

An esteemed group of top researchers from around the globe gathered to share their areas of expertise and interest and suggest some new strategies for improving athletes' ability to gain more from their training, recover more quickly from injury and perhaps experience fewer sick days. For example, while the latest evidence suggests that higher intake rates of carbohydrates during endurance competition can improve performance, the gut may need to be trained to tolerate this higher intake in the weeks leading up to a competition. On the contrary, some training bouts might best be undertaken at a relatively low carbohydrate intake and muscle status in order to extract greater training adaptations from the exercising muscle. Introducing the latest evidence and then discussing the ways to best integrate these nutritional strategies to ultimately help the athletes best prepare for their competitions is a great example of the raison d'être for the NNI sports nutrition-themed workshops.

We wish to express sincere gratitude to the chairpersons of this workshop, Prof. Luc J.C. van Loon and Prof. Kevin D. Tipton for creating an excellent theme and scientific program. We are also deeply indebted to the talented researchers who have furthered our understanding on this topic through their presentations and papers.

Finally, we want to thank Zibi Szlufcik and the PowerBar Europe Team as well as Natalia Wagemans of the Nestlé Nutrition Institute for the excellent logistical execution of the workshop in the magnificent setting of Majorca, Spain.

Eric Zaltas, MS, IOC Dipl Sports Nutrition
Global Head R&D, Performance Nutrition
Nestlé Nutrition

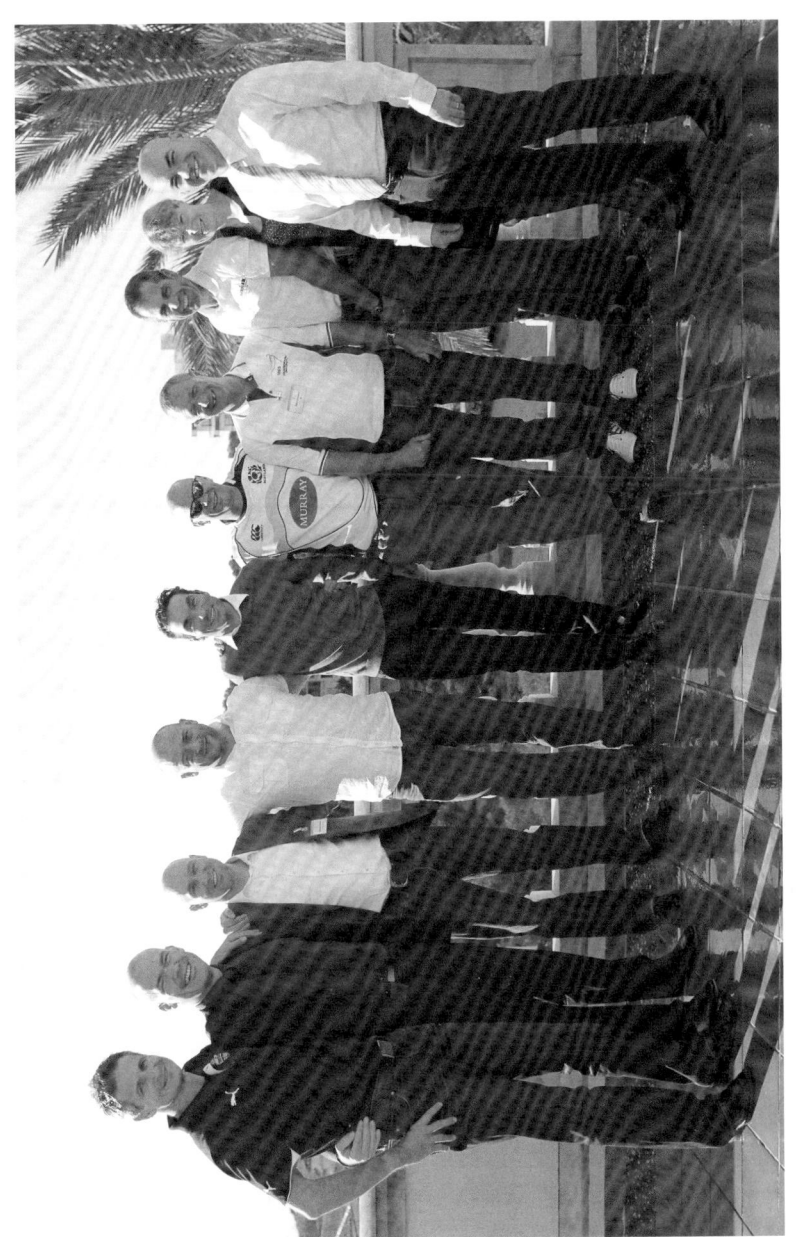

75th Nestlé Nutrition Institute Workshop
Mallorca, Spain, December 7–8, 2011

Contributors

Chairpersons & Speakers

Prof. Louise M. Burke
Sports Nutrition
Australian Institute of Sport
Leverrier Crescent
Bruce, ACT 2616
Australia
E-Mail: louise.burke@ausport.gov.au

Prof. Wim Derave
Department of Movement and
Sports Sciences
Ghent University
Watersportlaan 2
B–9000 Ghent
Belgium
E-Mail: wim.derave@ugent.be

Prof. Martin J. Gibala
Department of Kinesiology
McMaster University
1280 Main Street West
Hamilton, ON L8S 4K1
Canada
E-Mail: gibalam@mcmaster.ca

Prof. Michael Gleeson
School of Sport, Exercise and Health
Sciences
Loughborough University
Loughborough
Leicestershire LE11 3TU
UK
E-Mail: m.Gleeson@lboro.ac.uk

Prof. John A. Hawley
School of Medical Sciences
RMIT University
Plenty Road
Bundoora, VIC 3083
Australia
E-Mail: john.hawley@rmit.edu.au

Prof. Asker Jeukendrup
School of Sport and Exercise Sciences
University of Birmingham
Edgbaston
Birmingham B15 2TT
UK
E-Mail: a.e.jeukendrup@bham.ac.uk

Prof. Andrew M. Jones
Sport and Health Sciences,
University of Exeter
Exeter EX12LU
UK
E-Mail: a.m.jones@exeter.ac.uk

Dr. Enette Larson-Meyer
The University of Wyoming
Department 3354
1000 E. University Avenue
Laramie, WY 820 70
USA
E-Mail: enette@uwyo.edu

Prof. Melinda M. Manore
Oregon State University
Nutrition
School Biological and Population Health Sciences
Milam 103
Corvallis, OR 97331
USA
E-Mail: melinda.manore@oregonstate.edu

Prof. Kevin D. Tipton
School of Sport
University of Stirling
Stirling FK9 4LA
UK
E-Mail: k.d.tipton@stir.ac.uk

Prof. Luc J.C. van Loon
Department of Human Movement Sciences
Maastricht University Medical Centre+
PO Box 616
NL–6200 MD Maastricht
The Netherlands
E-Mail: L.vanLoon@maastrichtuniversity.nl

Nutritional Strategies to Modulate the Adaptive Response to Endurance Training

John A. Hawley

Exercise & Nutrition Research, School of Medical Sciences, RMIT University, Bundoora, VIC, Australia

Abstract

In recent years, advances in molecular biology have allowed scientists to elucidate how endurance exercise training stimulates skeletal muscle remodeling (i.e. promotes mitochondrial biogenesis). A growing field of interest directly arising from our understanding of the molecular bases of training adaptation is how nutrient availability can alter the regulation of many contraction-induced events in muscle in response to endurance exercise. Acutely manipulating substrate availability can exert profound effects on muscle energy stores and patterns of fuel metabolism during exercise, as well as many processes activating gene expression and cell signaling. Accordingly, such interventions when repeated over weeks and months have the potential to modulate numerous adaptive processes in skeletal muscle that ultimately drive the phenotype-specific characteristics observed in highly trained athletes. In this review, the molecular and cellular events that occur in skeletal muscle during and after endurance exercise are discussed and evidence provided to demonstrate that nutrient availability plays an important role in modulating many of the adaptive responses to training. Emphasis is on human studies that have determined the regulatory role of muscle glycogen availability on cell metabolism, endurance training capacity and performance.

Copyright © 2013 Nestec Ltd., Vevey/S. Karger AG, Basel

Introduction

The interaction between endurance exercise and nutrient availability has long been recognized, and it has generally been assumed that the optimal adaptation to the demands of repeated training sessions requires a diet that preserves muscle energy stores. The International Olympic Committee's Consensus Statement on Sports Nutrition published in 2003 reflected this paradigm and recommended that 'athletes should aim to achieve carbohydrate intakes to meet the fuel requirements of their training programme and to optimise restoration of muscle glycogen stores between workouts' [1]. In real life, however, competitive endurance athletes follow an intricate periodization of both diet and training load in their build-up to competition [2]. As such, the latest guidelines for the daily training environment acknowledge the complexity of these practices by encouraging 'strategies to promote carbohydrate availability for the *majority* of workouts as is practical and within the athletes total energy budget' [2, 3].

The field-based approaches of athletes are not without scientific basis: it has been hypothesized that a 'cycling' of muscle glycogen stores is essential to optimize training adaptation [4]. To this end, there has been recent interest in the systematic manipulation of muscle glycogen availability before and after selected training sessions and the subsequent effects on cell metabolism, training adaptation and performance. Such an approach is intended to form part of a periodized training program during which athletes intentionally commence specific workouts with either low muscle glycogen reserves and/or low exogenous carbohydrate availability [for reviews, see 5, 6]. Support for such a practice is slowly emerging: several investigations have reported that when endurance-based training sessions are commenced with low-glycogen availability, training adaptation is augmented to a greater extent than when similar workouts are undertaken with normal glycogen stores [5, 6]. What is apparent is that nutrient availability alters many training-induced skeletal muscle adaptations and could potentially be a valuable coaching strategy to modulate training efficiency. In this review, the molecular and cellular events that occur in skeletal muscle during and after endurance-based exercise are discussed and evidence provided to demonstrate that nutrient availability plays important roles in promoting many of the adaptive responses to training. Emphasis is on human studies that have determined the regulatory role of muscle glycogen availability on cell metabolism, endurance training capacity and performance. The reader is referred to several recent reviews for detailed discussion of other nutritional strategies that impact on training-induced skeletal muscle adaptations [2, 5, 6].

Training Adaptation

The key components of any endurance training program are the volume, intensity and frequency of exercise sessions, with the sum of these inputs being the 'training stimulus' that either promotes (fitness) or decreases (fatigue) performance capacity [7]. Modifications in skeletal muscle cells that persist as a consequence of training are termed chronic adaptations, whereas cellular alterations that occur in response to a single training session are said to be acute responses. Chronic adaptations in skeletal muscle are likely to be the result of the cumulative effect of repeated (acute) bouts of exercise, with the initial signaling responses leading to these adaptations occurring during recovery in each training session [8]. From a molecular perspective, training adaptation can be simplistically viewed as the accumulation of specific proteins (i.e. enzymes) with the increased gene expression promoting these changes in protein concentration pivotal to the adaptation process [9].

In recent years, advances in molecular biology have allowed scientists to determine how endurance exercise training stimulates mitochondrial biogenesis [for reviews, see 10–12]. The major breakthrough was the discovery of several transcription factors that regulate expression of the nuclear genes that encode mitochondrial proteins including nuclear-respiratory factor 1 (NRF-1) and NRF-2 which bind to the promoters and activate transcription of the genes that encode mitochondrial respiratory chain proteins [13]. NRF-1 also activates expression of the nuclear gene that encodes mitochondrial transcription factor A which moves to the mitochondria where it regulates transcription of the mitochondrial DNA (i.e. the mitochondrial genome). A second breakthrough was the discovery of an inducible coactivator, the peroxisome proliferator-activated receptor-γ coactivator (PGC-1α) that docks on and activates these transcription factors and, thus, activates and regulates the coordinated expression of mitochondrial proteins encoded in the nuclear and mitochondrial genomes [14]. A single bout of prolonged endurance exercise results in a rapid and sustained increase in PGC-1α protein expression [15] which is likely to be one of the mechanisms for modulating metabolic fluxes in skeletal muscle as a response to decreased ATP and altered fuel demands.

Another exercise-induced signal leading to increased mitochondrial biogenesis is the rise in muscle AMP concentration during exercise which activates the multi-substrate enzyme 5′-AMP-activated protein kinase (AMPK). AMPK functions as a metabolic 'fuel gauge' because when it becomes activated in response to decreased energy levels (i.e. muscle contraction), it inhibits ATP-consuming pathways and activates pathways involved in carbohydrate and fatty acid catabolism to restore ATP levels. The multi-faceted interaction of the AMPK with PGC-1α is likely to play a major role in both the acute responses and chronic exercise-induced adaptations in muscle [10, 11]. Finally, the p38 mitogen-activated protein kinase (p38 MAPK) can also phosphorylate and activate PGC-1α [16]. p38 MAPK increases PGC-1α expression by phosphorylating the transcription factor ATF-2, which increases PGC-1 protein expression by binding to and activating the CREB site on the PGC-1α promoter. Exercise results in rapid activation of p38 MAPK, which mediates both the activation and increased expression of PGC-1α [16]. The discovery of these (and other) major cell signaling pathways and their responses to exercise has allowed scientists to identify and characterize a range of muscle adaptations that appear to be specific to the modality of training (i.e. endurance- versus strength-based activities) and training history of the athlete [10, 17]. An emerging field of interest arising from our understanding of the molecular bases of training adaptation is how nutrient availability alters the regulation of many of the contraction-induced events in muscle in response to endurance-based exercise. Nutrient-gene and nutrient-protein interactions can promote or inhibit the activities of a number of cell signaling pathways and thereby modulate training adaptation and subsequent performance capacity.

Acute Effects of Altering Skeletal Muscle Carbohydrate Availability on Cell Metabolism

Skeletal muscle energy status exerts profound effects on resting fuel metabolism and patterns of fuel utilization during exercise as well as acute regulatory processes underlying gene expression and cell signaling [6]. In one of the first studies to investigate the regulatory role of muscle glycogen availability on cell metabolism, Wojtaszewski et al. [18] measured rates of fuel utilization and signaling responses in well-trained athletes who commenced a bout of submaximal cycling (60 min at 70% of peak O_2 uptake, VO_{2peak}) under conditions in which muscle glycogen content was manipulated by prior exercise and diet to be either low (~150 mmol/kg dry weight) or high (~900 mmol/kg dry weight). Based on respiratory exchange ratio values measured throughout exercise, the estimated contribution from carbohydrate to total energy expenditure was 10 ± 2 for the low- compared to 79 ± 1% for the high-glycogen condition ($p < 0.01$). Skeletal muscle biopsies from the vastus lateralis revealed similar concentrations of creatine phosphate and adenine nucleotides at rest, yet the activity of the AMPK and β-acetyl-CoA carboxylase Ser^{221} phosphorylation were lower in glycogen-loaded compared with glycogen-depleted muscles [18]. There were isoform-specific differences in AMPK activity in response to altered glycogen availability: resting AMPK-α1 activity was higher in the low- compared with the high-glycogen condition, but did not increase in response to exercise. In contrast, AMPK-α2 activity increased during exercise and was significantly higher during the low compared to the high glycogen trial ($p < 0.05$).

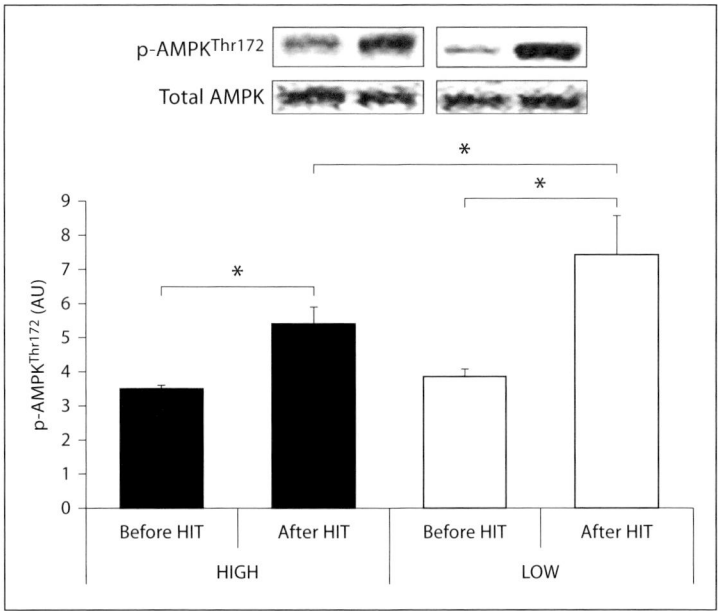

Fig. 1. Phosphorylation of AMPK (relative to total AMPK) at threonine 172 (p-AMPK^{Thr172}) before and after HIT commenced with either high (HIGH) or low (LOW) muscle glycogen concentration in two groups of endurance-trained cyclists/triathletes. HIGH (n = 6) performed a 100-min steady-state ride (AT) at ~70% of VO$_{2peak}$ on day 1 followed by HIT (8 × 5-min work bouts at maximal self-selected effort with 1-min recovery in between work bouts) 24 h later. LOW (n = 6) performed AT on day 1 at 08.00 h, and after 1–2 h of rest with no energy intake performed HIT. * $p < 0.05$, significantly different. Reproduced with permission from Yeo et al. [19].

Yeo et al. [19] recently reported that the magnitude of increase in AMPK phosphorylation in endurance-trained cyclists/triathletes who performed a bout of high-intensity interval training (HIT) was greater when the session was commenced with low compared to normal glycogen availability (fig. 1), while Steinberg et al. [20] found that increased activation of AMPK under conditions of low muscle glycogen availability enhanced AMPK-α$_2$ nuclear translocation in response to exercise in human skeletal muscle. Chan et al. [21] showed that commencing a bout of endurance exercise (60 min at 70% of VO$_{2peak}$) with low muscle glycogen availability resulted in a greater phosphorylation of the p38 MAPK at the nucleus compared to exercise commenced with normal glycogen levels. Several studies have reported a rapid induction of both PGC-1α mRNA [15, 22] and protein [15] following endurance exercise in humans, although glycogen availability has a negligible effect on the basal gene abundance of this transcription factor [23]. Taken collectively, these findings demonstrate that the basal activity and/or phosphorylation state and subsequent magnitude of exercise-induced activation of several key enzymes with putative roles in training adaptation are dependent on the fuel status of the muscle cells. The functional implications of these observations are likely to be important for the adaptive response to endurance training with regard to regulation of both metabolism and gene/protein expression.

Chronic Effects of Altering Skeletal Muscle Carbohydrate Availability on Cell Metabolism and Training Adaptation

Acute alterations in muscle glycogen availability alter the immediate exercise-induced response of a number of signaling pathways involved in the training response [18–21], and when repeated over weeks and months have the potential to modulate many adaptive processes in skeletal muscle and ultimately drive the phenotype-specific characteristics observed in highly trained athletes. In the first investigation to test this hypothesis, Hansen et al. [9] employed a study design in which the left and right legs of the same (untrained) individual undertook the same total work during a 10 week training intervention, albeit with different pre-exercise muscle glycogen availability for half the training sessions. These workers reported that resting muscle glycogen levels, the maximal activities of citrate synthase and exercise time to exhaustion were all enhanced to a greater extent in the leg that commenced half the workouts with low compared to normal glycogen availability.

To investigate whether competitive athletes with a prolonged history of endurance training might attain the same benefit as less fit individuals who undertake a training regimen with lowered glycogen availability, Yeo et al. [24] recruited competitive 12 male cyclists/triathletes and divided them into two groups matched for age, VO_{2peak} and training history. One group (HIGH) trained 6 days/week with one rest day (day 7) for 3 weeks, alternating between 100-min steady-state aerobic riding (AT; ~70% VO_{2peak}) on the first day and HIT (8 × 5-min work bouts at maximal effort with 1-min recovery in between work bouts at ~100 W) the next day. The AT and HIT sessions were deliberately chosen as both these workouts deplete ~50% of resting muscle glycogen stores in the fed state in well-nourished, trained athletes. The other group (LOW) trained twice a day, every 2nd day for 3 weeks, performing the AT in the morning to decrease muscle glycogen content, followed by ~2 h of rest without nutrient intake and then HIT. Accordingly, HIGH completed all HIT sessions at a time when muscle glycogen levels were restored, whereas LOW undertook this interval set at a time when muscle glycogen stores were 50% lower than normal. During week 1 (HIT sessions 1–3), LOW trained at a significantly lower average power output compared with HIGH ($p < 0.05$). During the 2nd week (HIT sessions 4–6), there was a trend for the average training intensity to be lower ($p = 0.06$), but by the 3rd week (HIT sessions 7–9), the training intensities between LOW and HIGH were not different. Resting muscle glycogen content, the maximal activities of citrate synthase and β-hydroxyacyl-CoA dehydrogenase and the content of the electron transport chain component COX subunit IV were all enhanced to a greater extent in LOW compared with HIGH after the 3 weeks' intervention. However, while markers of training adaptation were augmented when athletes trained LOW, the performance of a 1-hour time trial undertaken after a 60-min steady-state ride was similar after both training programs. These findings were subsequently confirmed by Hulston et al. [25]. While the term 'train low, compete high' has been used to describe the original twice-every-second-day protocol, a fact often overlooked is that in all of these investigations [9, 24, 25] subjects only performed half of their prescribed training sessions with low muscle glycogen availability.

Substrate Availability during Recovery from Endurance-Based Exercise

Recovery from endurance training is characterized by a multitude of changes in skeletal muscle cell metabolism that, depending on the intensity, duration and mode of the prior bout, can persist for many hours upon the cessation of exercise. For example, glucose uptake and glycogen synthase activity are highest in the first 2–3 h of recovery and reverse progressively as glycogen resynthesis takes place. The sensitivity of muscle to insulin is also dramatically increased during the initial recovery phase, being highest in the 1–2 h after exercise, progressively reversing as glycogen is restored [for review, see 26]. However, in situations in which muscle glycogen resynthesis is restricted or postponed (i.e. by delaying or withholding nutrient availability), muscle insulin sensitivity can remain elevated for up to 48 h [26]. The orchestrated pattern of these cellular events in muscle clearly demonstrates the high metabolic priority afforded to glycogen resynthesis during recovery from glycogen-depleting exercise [27].

There is a growing understanding that gene-specific transcriptional activation during and after a bout of exercise is involved in reestablishing cellular homeostasis in muscle in response to the prior exercise bout, as well as playing a major role in the adaptations that occur in response to exercise training. In this regard, a single bout of endurance exercise has been shown to increase mRNA expression of a large number of genes, the majority of which are involved in mitochondrial biogenesis and metabolism [28]. In addition, endurance exercise has been shown to elevate the mRNA expression of genes involved in oxidant stress management, electrolyte transport across membranes and extracellular matrix remodeling. Of interest here is whether substrate availability plays a major role in influencing the time course and magnitude of transcriptional activation and contributes to homeostatic recovery and adaptation.

Pilegaard et al. [27] performed two experiments to determine whether the magnitude and duration of exercise-induced transcription of 'metabolic genes' was influenced by pre-exercise muscle glycogen availability. In the first experiment, subjects performed one-legged cycling exercise (to lower glycogen content in one leg) and then, the following day completed 2–3 h of two-legged cycling. Biopsies were taken prior to and immediately after exercise and then at 2 and 5 h of recovery, during which subjects consumed foods high in carbohydrate. Before exercise, transcription of the pyruvate dehydrogenase kinase 4 (PDK4), uncoupling protein 3 (UCP3), hexokinase II (HKII) and lipoprotein lipase (LPL) genes was similar in legs with low or normal glycogen availability. However, in response to exercise, there was a significant increase in transcription of UCP3 only in the leg with low glycogen availability. Similar trends were observed for PDK4 and HKII. Transcription of all genes had returned to pre-exercise levels within 5 h after exercise. In a separate experiment, 6 subjects commenced two trials consisting of 3 h of two-legged knee extensor exercise with either low or normal glycogen availability. Biopsies were taken before exercise and throughout recovery in which no nutrients were provided. Low-glycogen availability affected the mRNA content of several genes prior to exercise including PDK4, UCP3 and HKII. In general, these differences persisted throughout exercise. During recovery, transcription of the PDK4 gene was significantly higher in the leg that commenced exercise with low glycogen availability (transcription for the UCP3, HKII or LPL genes was not determined).

Subsequently, these same workers studied subjects during recovery from a single bout of glycogen-depleting exercise when they consumed either a post-exercise diet high in carbohydrate and muscle glycogen availability was rapidly (within 5 h) restored to normal levels, or after a post-exercise diet low in carbohydrate diet when muscle glycogen availability remained depressed for 24 h [22]. Exercise increased the transcription and/or mRNA content of a number of genes with important roles in metabolism (including the PDK-4, UCP-3, LPL, HKII, carnitine palmitoyltransferase I, PGC-1α, and peroxisome proliferator activated receptor-α). Providing a high-carbohydrate diet during recovery (i.e. rapidly increasing muscle glycogen availability) resulted in a reversal in the activation of the majority of these genes within 5–8 h after exercise. In contrast, providing a low-carbohydrate diet during recovery (i.e. delaying muscle glyco-

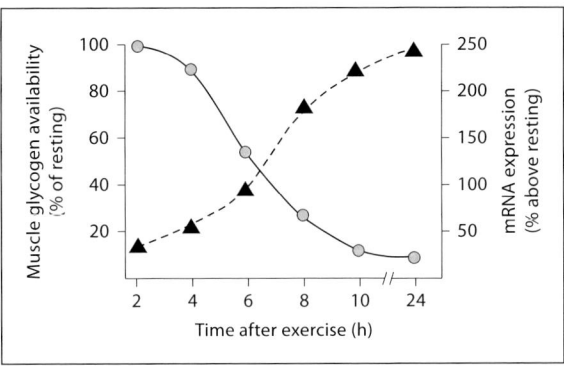

Fig. 2. Hypothetical schematic of the time course of the activity (mRNA expression) of 'exercise-induced metabolic genes' with putative roles in endurance training adaptation (grey circles) and the restoration of muscle glycogen stores (black triangles) following a single bout of prolonged, glycogen-depleting exercise. The activation of many exercise-induced genes peaks in the immediate hours of recovery (1–4 h) and has returned to basal levels within ~24 h of the last exercise bout. Low muscle glycogen availability enhances and prolongs the time course of transcriptional activation of many 'metabolic genes' in response to exercise (see text for discussion) raising the possibility that common signaling pathways sensitive to muscle glycogen availability and/or systematic factors (fatty acid availability and/or hormone levels) may be linked to the transcriptional control of these genes.

gen availability) elicited a sustained/enhanced increase in activation of these genes through 8–24 h of recovery. These findings [22, 27] demonstrate that factors associated with substrate availability (e.g. muscle glycogen restoration) influence the transcriptional regulation of metabolic genes in skeletal muscle of humans during recovery. The timing and transient nature of these differential gene responses raise the possibility that the regulation of transcription may be linked to common signaling mechanisms in the muscle that are sensitive to glycogen availability and/or systemic factors [27].

It should be noted that there is currently no evidence to support the notion that withholding carbohydrate during recovery from glycogen-depleting exercise promotes training adaptation to a greater extent than when glycogen stores are rapidly restored, although on theoretical grounds (fig. 2) this seems plausible. Current sport nutrition guidelines recommend that athletes achieve a total intake of carbohydrate commensurate with the fuel needs of their training sessions and promote the strategic intake of carbohydrate and protein before and after key training sessions to optimize the adaptations and enhance recovery [2, 3]. In this regard, the findings of Breen et al. [29] warrant discussion. These workers studied the responses of the different muscle proteins (mitochondrial and myofibrillar) in well-trained athletes during recovery from a bout of endurance cycling (90 min at 77% of VO_{2peak}) in which they ingested either carbohydrate (~25 g) or a carbohydrate (25 g) plus whey protein isolate (~10 g). Compared to the carbohydrate-only beverage, the carbohydrate-protein solution induced a rapid and sustained increase in serum insulin, plasma leucine and plasma threonine concentrations. The phosphorylation status of key enzymes with recognized roles in muscle growth was increased after 4 h of recovery only after ingestion of the carbohydrate-protein beverage. In accordance with these cell signaling responses, the authors demonstrated that coingestion of protein with carbohydrate enhanced the synthesis of the myofibrillar but not the mitochondrial protein fraction during recovery [29]. At first sight, these findings seem somewhat paradoxical: it is widely accepted that ingesting protein potentiates the 'anabolic' effect of resistance exercise by upregulating rates of myofibrillar protein synthesis. However, it may be that protein feeding after endurance exercise is important for maintaining the structural integrity and the power-generating capacity of the previously exercised musculature [29]. Alternatively, the mitochondrial protein fraction may be more of a priority later in the recovery period (i.e. to drive adaptive endurance responses) when amino acid availability is not limiting (i.e. after a meal). In support of this premise, Rowlands et al. [30] have reported that high protein intakes (~60 g) after prolonged (2.5 h) cycling initiate a transcriptional profile that favors the expression of genes involved in type I (slow-twitch) fiber remodeling and enhanced cellular energy pathways. Clearly, further work is necessary to determine the time course of post-transcriptional regulation, and if chronic post-exercise protein feedings are associated with functionally meaningful changes that promote an endurance-like phenotype.

Is 'Train Low' a Nutritional Strategy to Modulate Training Efficiency?

A direct outcome of any dietary periodization strategy is to perturb the training stimulus via manipulation of nutrient availability with the goal of augmenting training adaptation. However, a common finding when selected workouts are commenced with low glycogen availability is that athletes perform these sessions at a lower workload or intensity, largely because they perceive the effort to be higher, at least during the initial exposure to training low [24]. On average, the power outputs sustained during high-intensity workouts commenced with low glycogen availability are reduced by ~8% compared to when the same sessions are undertaken with normal or elevated glycogen availability [24, 25]. While such an outcome seems counterintuitive for the preparation of competitive athletes where high-intensity workouts are a critical component of a periodized training program, skeletal muscle markers of training adaptation are still augmented despite the lower 'training stimulus'. Accordingly, for competitive athletes unable to train daily but who can perform two workouts in close proximity, with the second session performed under conditions of low muscle glycogen availability, 'train low' may offer a time-efficient method of maintaining training adaptations and exercise capacity. One might also consider that 'train low' strategies could be used to accelerate the adaptation process in athletes recovering from an injury/illness, or who need to reach training milestones in a limited time frame. Of course, training with low glycogen availability may of itself be associated with reduced immune function, and the balance between adaptation (fitness) and breakdown (fatigue) needs to be considered on an individual basis.

'Train low' has now become a catchphrase in athletic circles as well as in the scientific literature. This terminology is frequently used to describe a range of practices other than the original protocol (i.e. commencing training sessions with low muscle glycogen availability) and as a generic or 'one-size-fits-all' theme promoted as a replacement to the era of the high-carbohydrate diet in sport [5]. However, there are many ways of achieving low carbohydrate availability before, during and after training sessions which differ in the site targeted for low carbohydrate availability (i.e. intra- vs. extra-muscular), in the duration of exposure, the number of tissues affected as well as the frequency and timing of their incorporation into an athlete's periodized training program. Finally, it needs to be stressed that many world-class endurance and ultra-endurance athletes already incorporate 'train low' strategies into their schedules and have done so for many years [Hawley, pers. commun.]. Prior to embarking on further lab-based investigations of 'train low', it may be beneficial to clarify whether successful athletes have already refined optimal nutrient-training protocols that enhance endurance performance and can better inform future scientific enquiry. Such an approach may ultimately result in scientists being in a better position to advise coaches about the optimal nutrient-exercise strategies that best modulate training efficiency.

Disclosure Statement

The author declares that no financial or other conflict of interest exists in relation to the content of the chapter.

References

1 Burke LM: The IOC consensus on sports nutrition 2003: new guidelines for nutrition for athletes. Int J Sport Nutr Exerc Metab 2003;13:549–552.
2 Burke LM: Fueling strategies to optimize performance: training high or training low? Scand J Med Sci Sports 2010;20(suppl 2): 48–58.
3 Burke LM, Hawley JA, Wong SH, Jeukendrup AE: Carbohydrates for training and competition. J Sports Sci 2011;29(suppl 1): S17–S27.
4 Chakravarthy MV, Booth FW: Eating, exercise, and 'thrifty' genotypes: connecting the dots toward an evolutionary understanding of modern chronic diseases. J Appl Physiol 2004;96:3–10.
5 Hawley JA, Burke LM: Carbohydrate availability and training adaptation: effects on cell metabolism. Exerc Sport Sci Rev 2010; 38:152–160.
6 Hawley JA, Burke LM, Phillips SM, Spriet LL: Nutritional modulation of training-induced skeletal muscle adaptations. J Appl Physiol 2011;110:834–845.
7 Hawley JA: Adaptations of skeletal muscle to prolonged, intense endurance training. Clin Exp Pharmacol Physiol 2002;29:218–222.
8 Pilegaard H, Ordway GA, Saltin B, Neufer PD: Transcriptional regulation of gene expression in human skeletal muscle during recovery from exercise. Am J Physiol Endocrinol Metab 2000;279:E806–E814.
9 Hansen AK, Fischer CP, Plomgaard P, et al: Skeletal muscle adaptation: training twice every second day vs training once daily. J Appl Physiol 2005;98:93–99.
10 Coffey VG, Hawley JA: The molecular bases of training adaptation. Sports Med 2007;37: 737–763.
11 Hawley JA, Holloszy JO: Exercise: it's the real thing! Nutr Rev 2009;67:172–178.
12 Kelly DP, Scarpulla RC: Transcriptional regulatory circuits controlling mitochondrial biogenesis and function. Genes Dev 2004;18: 357–368.
13 Scarpulla RC: Nuclear control of respiratory gene expression in mammalian cells. J Cell Biochem 2006;97:673–683.
14 Lin J, Handschin C, Spiegelman BM: Metabolic control through the PGC-1 family of transcription coactivators. Cell Metab 2005; 1:361–370.
15 Mathai AS, Bonen A, Benton CR, et al: Rapid exercise-induced changes in PGC-1alpha mRNA and protein in human skeletal muscle. J Appl Physiol 2008;105:1098–1105.
16 Akimoto T, Pohnert SC, Li P, et al: Exercise stimulates PGC-1α transcription in skeletal muscle through activation of the p38 MAPK pathway. J Biol Chem 2005;280:19587–19593.
17 Coffey VG, Shield A, Canny BJ, et al: Interaction of contractile activity and training history on mRNA abundance in skeletal muscle from trained athletes. Am J Physiol Endocrinol Metab 2006;290:E849–E855.
18 Wojtaszewski JF, MacDonald C, Nielsen JN, et al: Regulation of 5′AMP-activated protein kinase activity and substrate utilization in exercising human skeletal muscle. Am J Physiol Endocrinol Metab 2003;284:E813–E822.
19 Yeo WK, McGee SL, Carey AL, et al: Acute signalling responses to intense endurance training commenced with low or normal muscle glycogen. Exp Physiol 2010;95:351–358.
20 Steinberg GR, Watt MJ, McGee SL, et al: Reduced glycogen availability is associated with increased AMPKalpha2 activity, nuclear AMPK-α2 protein abundance, and GLUT4 mRNA expression in contracting human skeletal muscle. Appl Physiol Nutr Metab 2006;31:302–312.
21 Chan MH, McGee SL, Watt MJ, et al: Altering dietary nutrient intake that reduces glycogen content leads to phosphorylation of nuclear p38 MAP kinase in human skeletal muscle: association with IL-6 gene transcription during contraction. FASEB J 2004; 18:1785–1787.
22 Pilegaard H, Osada T, Andersen LT, et al: Substrate availability and transcriptional regulation of metabolic genes in human skeletal muscle during recovery from exercise. Metabolism 2005;54:1048–1055.
23 Pilegaard H, Saltin B, Neufer PD: Exercise induces transient transcriptional activation of the PGC-1α gene in human skeletal muscle. J Physiol 2003;546:851–858.
24 Yeo WK, Paton CD, Garnham AP, et al: Skeletal muscle adaptation and performance responses to once a day versus twice every second day endurance training regimens. J Appl Physiol 2008;105:1462–1470.

25 Hulston CJ, Venables MC, Mann CH, et al: Training with low muscle glycogen enhances fat metabolism in well-trained cyclists. Med Sci Sports Exerc 2010;42:2046–2055.
26 Holloszy JO: A forty-year memoir of research on the regulation of glucose transport into muscle. Am J Physiol Endocrinol Metab 2003;284:E453–E467.
27 Pilegaard H, Keller C, Steensberg A, et al: Influence of pre-exercise muscle glycogen content on exercise-induced transcriptional regulation of metabolic genes. J Physiol 2002;541:261–271.
28 Mahoney DJ, Parise G, Melov S, et al: Analysis of global mRNA expression in human skeletal muscle during recovery from endurance exercise. FASEB J 2005;19:1498–1500.
29 Breen L, Philp A, Witard OC, et al: The influence of carbohydrate-protein co-ingestion following endurance exercise on myofibrillar and mitochondrial protein synthesis. J Physiol 2011;589:4011–4025.
30 Rowlands DS, Thomson JS, Timmons BW, et al: Transcriptome and translational signaling following endurance exercise in trained skeletal muscle: impact of dietary protein. Physiol Genomics 2011;43:1004–1020.

Questions and Answers

Question 1: So Dr. Hawley, exercising on low glycogen content stimulates fat oxidation; are there any further benefits to doing this?

Answer: Well, yes, there are several other adaptations in the muscle which tend to promote training adaptation to a greater extent than when you train with normal muscle glycogen content. These include the upregulation of key enzymes involved in mitochondrial biogenesis and fuel substrate handling. However, I think the emphasis on the increased rates of fat oxidation has been overplayed: most endurance-based events oxidize predominately carbohydrate, and are reliant on this fuel for the majority of skeletal muscle energy provision. Although we can increase fat oxidation dramatically, in almost all the studies so far reported (with one single exception) we have been unable to detect any performance improvement from this extra capacity to oxidize fat. So, yes, you can burn extra fat and give the muscle more capacity to generate energy from this source, but this does not appear to translate into useful improvements in athletic performance.

Question 2: What are the disadvantages of training with low muscle glycogen content?

Answer: Well, at the moment, the published studies have only been undertaken for a maximum of 10 weeks, so we have not detected any deleterious effects on health outcomes or other measures within the muscle. But my guess is that if you train chronically (i.e. for several months) on a very low carbohydrate diet, you may be more prone to disturbances in immune function, and maybe a greater incidence of illness or injuries. But again, that evidence is not out there yet because the majority of the studies have only used very short intervention periods. The bottom line is that the 'train low' approach is only one part of a general periodized exercise-nutrition plan, and not the sole form of training!

Question 3: Based on the train low principle, would it be better to train in the morning prior to breakfast?

Answer: Certainly training in the morning after an overnight fast and with low carbohydrate availability, either low muscle glycogen or low exogenous carbohydrate availability would shift the balance from carbohydrate to fat-based fuels. There is absolutely no question about that whatsoever.

Question 4: Can you also train over long periods with low glycogen content?

Answer: Well, although low glycogen increases fat metabolism, the problem with only using fat for a fuel for the muscle is that the intensity of the exercise has to be reduced. So, yes, you may be able to train over a long duration, but for the competitive athlete, if the training intensity is compromised then that is unlikely to result in a greater adaptation or performance.

Question 5: What would you recommend for athletes who wish to lose bodyweight?

Answer: That is a good question. There is certainly evidence to show that if you train with low carbohydrate availability (endogenous and/or exogenous availability), rates of whole-body fat oxidation will be increased compared to training with normal (or elevated) carbohydrate availability. If you want to use more fat (e.g. want to make weight for a competition), training with low glycogen availability could promote some of those adaptations to enhance greater fat utilization.

Question 6: So, would you also recommend to athletes to do high-intensity interval training combined with a low-carbohydrate diet?

Answer: Well, the studies we have performed certainly show that when you train with low muscle carbohydrate availability, your maximal self-selected training intensity is compromised by approximately 7–8% compared with performing the same session with normal glycogen status. On the other hand, when you look at adaptations in the muscle some of the training-induced adaptations are actually amplified. So, I guess it's a trade-off: you train at a lower intensity that the coach or athlete might be comfortable with, but as far as the things that we as exercise physiologists can measure in the lab, we think it gives the muscle adaptations which, in theory at least, should lead to enhanced performance.

Question 7: Would you recommend athletes to consume protein before exercising?

Answer: No, there is no evidence at the moment to show that protein ingestion before endurance type exercise has any benefit whatsoever. The role for protein is during post-exercise recovery.

Practical Considerations for Bicarbonate Loading and Sports Performance

Louise M. Burke

Sports Nutrition, Australian Institute of Sport, Bruce, ACT, Australia

Abstract

Consumption of sodium bicarbonate (300 mg/kg 1–2 h before exercise) can temporarily increase blood bicarbonate concentrations, enhancing extracellular buffering of hydrogen ions which accumulate and efflux from the working muscle. Such 'bicarbonate loading' provides an ergogenic strategy for sporting events involving high rates of anaerobic glycolysis which are otherwise limited by the body's capacity to manage the progressive increase in intracellular acidity. Studies show that bicarbonate loading strategies have a moderate positive effect on the performance of sports involving 1–7 min of sustained strenuous exercise, and may also be useful for prolonged sports involving intermittent or sustained periods of high-intensity work rates. This potential to enhance sports performance requires further investigation using appropriate research design, but may be limited by practical considerations such as gut discomfort or the logistics of the event. The effect of chronic use of bicarbonate supplementation prior to high-intensity workouts to promote better training performance and adaptations is worthy of further investigation. While this relatively simple dietary strategy has been studied and used by sports people for over 80 years, it is likely that there are still ways in which further benefits from bicarbonate supplementation can be developed and individualized for specific athletes or specific events. Copyright © 2013 Nestec Ltd., Vevey/S. Karger AG, Basel

Introduction

Bicarbonate is an extracellular anion with important roles in maintaining pH and electrolyte gradients between intra- and extracellular environments. Consumption of large amounts of bicarbonate can temporarily increase blood bicarbonate concentrations and pH, enhancing extracellular capacity to dispose of hydrogen ions which accumulate and efflux from the working muscle [1]. Such 'bicarbonate loading' provides an ergogenic strategy for sporting events involving high rates of anaerobic glycolysis which are otherwise limited by the body's capacity to manage the progressive increase in intracellular acidity. Although the direct role of hydrogen ion accumulation in muscle fatigue is unclear [2], there is evidence dating back to the 1930s that dietary strategies that decrease blood pH (e.g. intake of acid salts) impair the capacity for high-intensity exercise, while alkalotic therapies such as the intake of bicarbonate improve such performance [3]. This review provides an update on the practical issues involved in bicarbonate loading for sports performance and raises questions that are as yet unanswered.

Acute Loading Protocols

The most common bicarbonate loading technique is to ingest an acute dose in the hours before the targeted exercise session. Ideally, sufficient bicarbonate is consumed at the optimal time to create a meaningful increase in blood bicarbonate concentrations and buffering capacity. A cheap and widely available form of bicarbonate is the common household/cooking product, sodium bicarbonate, with the typical dose being 300 mg per kg of the athlete's body mass (BM; i.e. ~20 g for a 70-kg athlete) consumed 1–2 h prior to exercise. Many athletes find, however, that a mixture of 4–5 tsp of sodium bicarbonate in water or other fluids is unpalatably salty. Alternative options include pharmaceutical alkalizer products: powders, capsules or tablets which have been developed to relieve the discomfort associated with urinary tract infections. Citrate has also been used as a buffering agent. However, since it appears to be less effective in enhancing performance and is associated with a greater risk of side effects [4], it will not be discussed further in this review.

The major side effect of bicarbonate supplementation is gastrointestinal (GI) distress including nausea, stomach pain, diarrhea and vomiting [1]. Indeed, sports scientists often observe that bicarbonate loading is not practiced by athletes who could potentially benefit from an enhanced buffering capacity in a competitive setting due to the fear or personal experience of such GI upsets. Previous advice to athletes to overcome this issue was to consume the bicarbonate dose with plenty of fluids to reduce the risk of hyperosmotic diarrhea. A recent study systematically investigated bicarbonate supplementation protocols, varying the time taken to consume the load (spreading it over 30–60 min), the form of the bicarbonate (flavored powder or capsules) and the coingestion of various amounts of fluid or food with the bicarbonate [5]. The strategy that optimized blood alkalosis and reduced the occurrence of GI symptoms was to consume bicarbonate capsules in a spread-out protocol, commencing 120–150 min before the start of exercise and, if practical, at the same time as consuming a meal composed of carbohydrate-rich food choices and some fluid. Athletes should practice with such strategies to fine-tune a successful protocol for their situation [5].

Even if gut issues can be overcome, athletes should consider the potential for other practical problems associated with bicarbonate loading. Loading with sodium bicarbonate involves the intake of a large amount of sodium, which when consumed with fluid can lead to a temporary fluid retention or hyperhydration. This may be useful in some sports in which high rates of sweat loss will otherwise lead to a significant fluid deficit. On the other hand, the gain in BM may be unwelcome to athletes in weight-bearing sports or weight-category sports. Another potential disadvantage of bicarbonate loading is when the athlete is selected for a post-event doping test. Although bicarbonate loading is a legal strategy in competitive sport, it can produce urine with a pH that falls outside the range that is acceptable for laboratory testing. The athlete may be required to wait several hours before he/she can produce a urine sample with pH levels that are acceptable to drug testing authorities. This may cause some disruption to the athlete's recovery routines.

Benefits for Sports Performance

Theoretically, bicarbonate loading could be ergogenic for sporting events which are limited by high rates of generation of energy via anaerobic glycolysis. The obvious candidates are events involving sustained high-intensity exercise lasting 1–7 min ('sustained power' sports), such as middle-distance swimming, middle-distance running and rowing events. However, bicarbonate loading may also benefit the performance of longer events (e.g. 30–60 min) involving sustained exercise just below the so-called anaerobic threshold if it can support the athlete for periods in which the pace is increased (i.e. surges during the event, the final sprint to the end). Similarly, the repeated-sprint performance typical of team and racquet sports, and even combative sports, may also be enhanced by improved buffering.

Over the past 40 years, sports scientists have investigated this potential in a large number of studies with various levels of application to real-life sport. Ideally, research that is of interest to athletes would involve highly trained competitors, exercise protocols with high reliability and ecological validity, and implementation of competition nutrition strategies that simulate real-world practices [6]. Although few studies achieve all these characteristics, table 1 summarizes the results of some relevant investigations of bicarbonate supplementation and sports performance published in the last decade. This summary shows that there is reasonable but not unanimous support for the benefits of bicarbonate loading for each of the sporting scenarios previously mentioned.

Nevertheless, reviews of the larger body of literature have concluded in different ways that bicarbonate loading can be of benefit to some athletes, particularly the so-called power events. An early meta-analysis [7] concluded that the ingestion of sodium bicarbonate has a moderate positive effect on exercise of 30 s to 7 min, with the mean performance of the bicarbonate trial being 0.44 standard deviations better than the placebo trial. Ergogenic effects were related to the level of metabolic acidosis achieved during the exercise, showing the importance of attaining a threshold pH gradient across the cell membrane from the combination of the accumulation of intracellular H^+ and the extracellular alkalosis. Requena et al. [8] undertook a narrative review which concluded that athletes competing in high-intensity sports involving fast motor unit activity and large muscle mass recruitment (athletics events, cycling, rowing, swimming and many team sports) could benefit from bicarbonate loading.

Finally, a recent comprehensive meta-analysis [4] of 38 studies and 137 estimates of the effect of blinded sodium bicarbonate supplementation on exercise outcomes quantified the mean effects of performance. It found a possibly moderate performance enhancement of 1.7% (90% confidence limit ± 2.0%) with a typical dose of ~0.3 g/kg BM) in a single 1-min sprint in male athletes. Study and subject characteristics had the following modifying small effects: an increase of 0.5% (±0.6%) with a 0.1 mg/kg BM increase in dose; an increase of 0.6% (±0.4%) with five extra sprint bouts; a reduction of 0.6% (±0.9%) for each 10-fold increase in test duration (e.g. 1–10 min); reductions of 1.1% (±1.1%) with non-athletes and 0.7% (±1.4%) with females. The only noteworthy effects involving physiological variables were a small correlation between performance and pre-exercise increase in blood bicarbonate [4].

Alternative Ways to Use Bicarbonate in Sport

A variation of the acute loading regime is to 'serially' load bicarbonate in small doses over consecutive days prior to a competitive event or race. Initial studies demonstrated that several days of such dosing (500 mg/kg BM spread into 3–4 separate doses over the day) builds up blood buffer levels that persist for at least 24 h after the last dose and with fewer gut symptoms [9]. Theoretically, this protocol could be used to achieve a loading preparation for multiple events over the

Table 1. Crossover studies of acute bicarbonate supplementation prior to sports-specific performance test in trained individuals (2002–2012)

Subjects and study	Dose of sodium bicarbonate	Sports performance	Enhancement	Comments
8 highly trained male swimmers [11]	300 mg/kg per day 105–90 min before trial	Swimming 200-meter TT followed by a further TT 24 h later	Immediate TT – no TT 24 h later – no	No enhancement of TT performance compared with placebo (1:59.57 ± 0:06.21 vs. 1:59.02 ± 0:05.82) and no difference in further TT after 24 h suggested that highly trained athletes may already have enhanced muscle buffering capacity and benefit less from bicarbonate loading.
10 elite moto-cross (BMX) cyclists [12]	300 mg/kg 90 min before trial	BMX simulation 3 × 30-second cycling Wingate tests with 15-min recovery Counter movement jump	No No	Authors concluded that test protocol may not have produced sufficient H^+ efflux to benefit from additional buffering.
8 well-trained rowers [13]	300 mg/kg and/or 6 mg/kg caffeine before trial	Rowing 2,000-meter ergometer TT	No	Performance was enhanced by ~2% with caffeine, but GI symptoms associated with bicarbonate counteracted this leading to unclear performance outcome.
20 male cyclists [14] Parallel group design for β-alanine with crossover for bicarbonate	300 mg/kg before trial and/or 4 weeks at 6.4 g/day β-alanine	Cycling TTE at 110% power max	Perhaps	β-Alanine enhanced cycling capacity. Addition of bicarbonate increased TTE by 6 s (4% increase), which did not reach statistical significance, but according to magnitude-based inferences has a 70% probability of being a meaningful improvement.
25 male rugby players [15]	300 mg/kg 65 min before warm-up	Rugby Union Rugby-specific repeated sprint test after 25-min warm-up + 9-min rugby-specific play	No	No difference in performance of rugby-specific test between trials. High risk of gut side effects reported that may impair performance.
9 collegiate male tennis players [16]	300 mg/kg before and 100 mg/kg during exercise	Tennis Simulated tennis match with Loughborough Tennis skill test performed before and after	Yes	Consistency scores for a number of strokes declined significantly after match with placebo, but were maintained in the bicarbonate trial.
12 elite female water polo players [17]	300 mg/kg before exercise	Water polo 59-min match simulation with 56 × 10-meter sprint swims	No	Percentage difference in mean sprint times with bicarbonate vs. placebo was not substantial (0.4 ± 1.0, $p = 0.51$).
10 male amateur boxers [18]	300 mg/kg before exercise	Boxing Sparring: 4 × 3-min rounds with 1-min recovery	Yes	Significant increase in punches successfully landed in bicarbonate trial.
6 male and 8 female competitive swimmers [19]	300 mg/kg before exercise	Swimming 8 × 25 m with 5-second recovery (simulation of 200-meter race controlled for variability in turns)	Yes	Total swim time was 2% faster in the bicarbonate trial (159.4 ± 25.4 vs. 163.2 ± 25.6 s; $p < 0.04$).

Table 1. Continued

Subjects and study	Dose of sodium bicarbonate	Sports performance	Enhancement	Comments
6 elite male swimmers [20]	300 mg/kg spread 120–30 min before trial 6 mg/kg caffeine 45 min before trial	Swimming 2 × 200-meter TT on 30-min recovery	No, for a one-off 200-meter TT Yes, for repeat 200-meter TTs	Bicarbonate enhanced performance, with and without caffeine on repeat performance. Effect was less evident for a single effort.
9 elite male BMX riders [21]	300 mg/kg 90 min before trial	BMX simulation 3 × 30-second cycling Wingate tests with 30-min recovery	No	Authors concluded that test protocol may have been too short and recovery period too long to sufficiently challenge buffering capacity.
9 elite male swimmers [22]	300 mg/kg spread 90–60 min before trial	Swimming 200-meter TT	Yes	Swimming TT with bicarbonate trial was 1.6% faster than placebo trial in internationally competitive swimmers.
4 female and 12 male national level endurance runners [23]	300 mg/kg 120–90 min before trial	Running 1,000-meter track run	Perhaps – but due to belief effect?	Fastest run when told and received bicarbonate (184.7 ± 24.1 s) with next best time when told they had received active agent but did not receive it (185.1 ± 22.1 s). Times when told no active agent were similar despite receiving bicarbonate (188.5 ± 24.4 s) or not (187.9 ± 22.4 s). Overall, the only statistically significant effect was a main effect of being told they had received an active agent.
9 national level judo athletes [24] 14 national level judo athletes	300 mg/kg 120 min before trial 300 mg/kg 120 min before trial	Judo Three judo-specific throwing fitness tests on 5-min recovery Four Wingate anaerobic upper body tests on 3-min recovery	Yes Yes	Bicarbonate supplementation increased total throws completed, primarily in bouts two and three. Greater mean power with bicarbonate supplementation in bouts three and four and greater PPO in bout four.
7 female team sports players [25]	2 × 200 mg/kg 90 and 20 min before exercise	Team sport simulation Intermittent cycling protocol of 2 × 36-min 'halves' involving repeated 2-min blocks (all out 4-second sprint, 100-second active recovery at 35% $VO_{2\,peak}$, and 20 s of rest)	Yes	Bicarbonate supplementation failed to produce any effect on performance in first half, but caused trend towards improved total work in the second half ($p = 0.08$). In particular, subjects completed significantly more work in 7 of 18 4-second sprints in second half in the bicarbonate trial.
15 competitive male distance runners [26]	300 mg/kg 90–180 min before race	Running Treadmill run to exhaustion at speed designed to last 1–2 min	Yes	Analysis estimated likelihood of treatments increasing endurance compared to placebo by at least 0.5% (smallest worthwhile improvement). Bicarbonate produced 2.7% enhancement of endurance (96% chance of improvement)

Table 1. Continued

Subjects and study	Dose of sodium bicarbonate	Sports performance	Enhancement	Comments
8 male + 8 female national level swimmers [27] (30-day washout)	300 mg/kg, 120 min before exercise (6 days at 20 g/day creatine also taken prior to bicarbonate trial)	Swimming 2 × 100-meter swims with 10-meter passive recovery	Yes (?)	Faster time for second swim with creatine/bicarbonate trial than with placebo: 1-second reduction in performance from first swim in placebo compared with 0.1-second drop-off in supplement trial ($p < 0.05$). Study unable to indicate individual effect of bicarbonate.
8 active male runners [28]	300 mg/kg 1 h before exercise	Team sport simulation: Intermittent cycling protocol of 30 min involving repeated 3-minute blocks (90 s at 40%, 60 s at 60% $VO_{2\,max}$ and 14 s at maximal sprint)	Yes	Significant main effect with greater PPO achieved in 14-second sprints across protocol in bicarbonate trial, whereas placebo trial showed gradual decline in PPO across time. Blood lactate levels higher than is generally reported in team sports; thus, movement patterns may not reflect the true workloads or physiological limitations of team sports.
7 female and 3 male collegiate swimmers [29] Dose-response design	100, 200 or 300 mg/kg 60 min before TT (45 min before warm-up)	Swimming 100- to 400-meter TT depending on main event, short course pool	Yes at all doses	Swimmers improved TT performances at all doses: compared with control, times were 97.0 ± 1.27% for 0.1 g/kg, 98.19 ± 1.75% for 0.2 g/kg and 99.10 ± 1.02% for 0.3 g/kg, all $p < 0.05$. Side effects increased with increasing dose.
6 well-trained male cyclists/triathletes and 1 cross-country skier [30]	300 mg/kg 2 h before exercise	Cycling 30 min at 77% $VO_{2\,max}$ + TT (~30 min)	No	Increase in blood lactate but no difference in TT performance time, muscle glycogen utilization or lactate.

Adapted from Burke et al. [6] with studies listed in reverse chronological order of date of publication. LT = Lactate threshold; PO = power output; PPO = peak power output; TT = time trial.

same/successive days or to time doses to avoid high-risk periods for gut upsets (i.e. acutely before, or even day of, exercise). Unfortunately, there are few studies of the effectiveness of this protocol on sports performance, and investigations in trained individuals are welcomed.

Another line of investigation is the chronic use of bicarbonate to support the training process rather than competition performance. Edge et al. [10] studied the effects of chronically loading with bicarbonate (400 mg/kg BM) prior to interval training sessions (3/week) over an 8-week training block in moderately trained female athletes. The bicarbonate-supplemented group showed substantially greater improvements in both lactate threshold (26 vs. 15%) and time to exhaustion (164 vs. 123%) than a placebo group. The authors speculated that training intensity rather than accumulation of hydrogen ions is important in increasing endogenous muscle buffering capacity, and that buffering protocols may reduce damage to muscle proteins [11]. This also warrants further investigation.

Conclusions

Although there is a large body of literature spanning nearly 80 years which shows general support for the use of bicarbonate loading to aid performance of sustained high-intensity sports, there are still many questions or issues that require clarification and further investigation:

1. Best protocols for acute (or serial) bicarbonate loading to enhance blood buffering capacity and minimize the risk of GI upsets.
2. Individual variability in the response to bicarbonate loading in trained individuals: effect of caliber of athlete, training history, sex, practice to develop gut tolerance.
3. Protocols to accommodate warm-up involving high-intensity pieces or longer event interspersed with high-intensity periods and repeated sprints.
4. Protocols to accommodate events with several bouts in a short period, for example several races on the same program or heats/semis/finals within 6–24 h.
5. Combination with other evidence-based supplements – e.g. caffeine, nitrate, creatine, β-alanine. Are the benefits additive, counteractive or synergistic?
6. Chronic application of bicarbonate loading to enhance training adaptations to interval training.

Disclosure Statement

The author has no conflicts of interest.

References

1 McNaughton LR, Siegler J, Midgley A: Ergogenic effects of sodium bicarbonate. Curr Sports Med Rep 2008;7:230–236.
2 Sahlin K: Metabolic factors in fatigue. Sports Med 1992;13:99–107.
3 Dennig H, Talbot JH, Edwards HT, et al: Effects of acidosis and alkalosis upon the capacity for work. J Clin Invest 1931;9:601–613.
4 Carr AJ, Slater GJ, Gore CJ, et al: Effect of sodium bicarbonate on [HCO3–], pH, and gastrointestinal symptoms. Int J Sport Nutr Exerc Metab 2011;21:189–194.
5 Carr AJ, Hopkins WG, Gore CJ: Effects of acute alkalosis and acidosis on performance: a meta-analysis. Sports Med 2011;41:801–814.
6 Burke L, Broad E, Cox G, et al: Supplements and sports foods; in Burke L, Deakin V (ed): Clinical Sports Nutrition, ed 4. Sydney, McGraw Hill, 2010, pp 419–500.
7 Matson LG, Tran ZT: Effects of sodium bicarbonate ingestion on anaerobic performance: a meta-analytic review. Int J Sport Nutr 1993;3:2–28.
8 Requena B, Zabala M, Padial P, et al: Sodium bicarbonate and sodium citrate: ergogenic aids? J Strength Cond Res 2005;19:213–224.
9 McNaughton L, Backx K, Palmer G, et al: Effects of chronic bicarbonate ingestion on the performance of high-intensity work. Eur J Appl Physiol 1999;80:333–336.
10 Edge J, Bishop D, Goodman C: Effects of chronic NaHCO3 ingestion during interval training on changes to muscle buffer capacity, metabolism and short-term endurance performance. J Appl Physiol 2006;101:918–925.
11 Joyce S, Minahan C, Anderson M, et al: Acute and chronic loading of sodium bicarbonate in highly trained swimmers. Eur J Appl Physiol 2012;112:461–469.
12 Zabala M, Requena B, Sánchez-Muñoz C, et al: Effects of sodium bicarbonate ingestion on performance and perceptual responses in a laboratory-simulated BMX cycling qualification series. J Strength Cond Res 2008;22:1645–1653.
13 Carr AJ, Gore CJ, Dawson B: Induced alkalosis and caffeine supplementation: effects on 2,000-m rowing performance. Int J Sport Nutr Exerc Metab 2011;21:357–364.
14 Sale C, Saunders B, Hudson S, et al: Effect of β-alanine plus sodium bicarbonate on high-intensity cycling capacity. Med Sci Sports Exerc 2011;43:1972–1978.
15 Cameron SL, McLay-Cooke RT, Brown RC, et al: Increased blood pH but not performance with sodium bicarbonate supplementation in elite rugby union players. Int J Sport Nutr Exerc Metab 2010;20:307–321.
16 Wu CL, Shih MC, Yang CC, et al: Sodium bicarbonate supplementation prevents skilled tennis performance decline after a simulated match. J Int Soc Sports Nutr 2010;7:33.
17 Tan F, Polglaze T, Cox G, et al: Effects of induced alkalosis on simulated match performance in elite female water polo players. Int J Sport Nutr Exerc Metab 2010;20:198–205.
18 Siegler JC, Hirscher K: Sodium bicarbonate ingestion and boxing performance. J Strength Cond Res 2010;24:103–108.
19 Siegler JC, Gleadall-Siddall DO: Sodium bicarbonate ingestion and repeated swim sprint performance. J Strength Cond Res 2010;24:3105–3111.
20 Pruscino CL, Ross ML, Gregory JR, et al: Effects of sodium bicarbonate, caffeine and their combination on repeated 200-m freestyle performance. Int J Sport Nutr Exerc Metab 2008;18:116–130.
21 Zabala M, Peinado AB, Calderón FJ, et al: Bicarbonate ingestion has no ergogenic effect on consecutive all out sprint tests in BMX elite cyclists. Eur J Appl Physiol 2011;111:3127–3134.
22 Lindh AM, Peyrebrune MC, Ingham SA, et al: Sodium bicarbonate improves swimming performance. Int J Sports Med 2008;29:519–523.
23 McClung M, Collins D: Because I know it will: placebo effects of an ergogenic aid on athletic performance. J Sport Exerc Psych 2007;29:383–394.
24 Artioli GG, Gualano B, Coelho DF, et al: Does sodium-bicarbonate ingestion improve simulated judo performance? Int J Sport Nutr Exerc Metab 2007;17:206–217.

25 Bishop D, Claudius B: Effects of induced metabolic alkalosis on prolonged intermittent-sprint performance. Med Sci Sports Exerc 2005;37:759–767.
26 Montfoort MCE, Van Dieren L, Hopkins WG, et al: Effects of ingestion of bicarbonate, citrate, lactate, and chloride on sprint running. Med Sci Sports Exerc 2004;36:1239–1243.
27 Mero AA, Keskinen KL, Malvela MT, et al: Combined creatine and sodium bicarbonate supplementation enhances interval swimming. J Strength Cond Res 2004;18:306–310.
28 Price M, Moss P, Rance S: Effects of sodium bicarbonate ingestion on prolonged intermittent exercise. Med Sci Sports Exerc 2003;38:1303–1308.
29 Bowman SA: The Effect of Different Dosing Strategies of Sodium Bicarbonate upon Collegiate Swimmers. Eugene, University of Oregon, 2002.
30 Stephens TJ, McKenna MJ, Canny BJ, et al: Effect of sodium bicarbonate on muscle metabolism during intense endurance cycling. Med Sci Sports Exerc 2002;34:614–621.

Questions and Answers

Question 1: So Dr. Burke, what side effects can be expected from using bicarbonate prior to competition?

Answer: Well, many athletes have unfortunate side effects in the form of gut problems that can range from burping and feeling a little bit squeamish in the stomach right through to vomiting and diarrhea. This is not a good look and may also be performance impairing.

Question 2: Is there a benefit to using sodium bicarbonate as a training aid?

Answer: It could be useful to try and support the training session to allow the athlete to train harder, but also to reduce some of the negative side effects of having a high acidity in the muscle so you may get less damage to the muscle and a better training outcome in the long-term.

Question 3: So what is your practical recommendation for athletes to use this substance?

Answer: It's tricky as we have changed our mind over the last 5–10 years. We think there is probably room for doing it in competition as long as the athlete can practice with it and learn to tolerate the gastric side effects. The training side of things has good hypothetical support, but it is a bit messy and logistically difficult for an athlete to bicarb load before many individual training sessions, so maybe looking for a more chronically applied buffer for the training support is a better way to go.

Question 4: A lot of athletes are now using β-alanine. What do you think about this?

Answer: That's the chronically applied buffer I was talking about. It's a supplement that can improve the muscle's internal buffering capacity by chronically increasing muscle stores of the cellular buffer carnosine. Once loading has been achieved it could assist each training session. On competition day, you could also consider adding bicarbonate loading. This could result in both the internal and external buffering system being improved, and the combined outcome could be beneficial.

Question 5: Is there a specific amount which you recommend for athletes if they use the sodium bicarbonate and β-alanine?

Answer: When we are working with bicarbonate, the typical dose is around 300 mg or 0.3 g for every kg of body weight; for me it would be something like 15 g of bicarbonate, for a 70-kg athlete about 20 g, which is quite a large dose. But we certainly play around with that because there are different ways in which athletes might need to use it, particularly if you are in a sport in which you might need to compete more than once. So, if you've got heats and finals of an event, you might use one dose for the first application, and then you might need to alter the dose for the second application. It's one of those things that are important to work through with a sports scientist in training, so that you can get the protocol that works right for you in competition.

Question 6: What about β-alanine?

Answer: β-Alanine is a chronically consumed supplement; something that you take every day and our initially used doses were about 3–4 g per day, for 10 weeks. We now think you can achieve a faster loading with 6–8 g per day for 4 weeks, then perhaps reduce it to 2 or 3 g per day. Ideally, spread you should those doses out over the day and use sustained-release formulations, so that you'd get the minimization of the prickly sensation that can happen when you take a β-alanine, supplement.

Question 7: Is β-alanine of relevance for athletes like weightlifters, or just for endurance sports?

Answer: It's important for athletes doing high-intensity work, where there's an accumulation of the hydrogen ions, and the acidity builds up in the muscle. That could be for people doing intermittent high intensity work or doing single sessions at sustained high intensities for 2–8 min. For many athletes, training will incorporate those sort of session; so, it could be a training aid for a whole range of sports as well as for those athletes that deal with the very high intensity work as their sporting performance outcome.

Question 8: What is the difference between creatine and β-alanine because a lot of studies are now using both supplements? What's the benefit or why do they combine both supplements?

Answer: When you take creatine as a supplement, you build up the phosphocreatine stores in the muscle which provide a fuel source for exercise. β-alanine supplemetation is trying to build up muscle carnosine, which may, help your ability to exercise for longer before the muscle starts to fatigue. Thus, in one case you've got a fuel, and in the other case you've got the environment that allows muscle fuel to be used at high intensities for a longer period. Of course we are also beginning to lean that muscle carnosine has other important activities that could also enhance exercise performance. Future studies may identify new benefits.

Influence of Dietary Nitrate Supplementation on Exercise Tolerance and Performance

Andrew M. Jones · Anni Vanhatalo · Stephen J. Bailey

Sport and Health Sciences, College of Life and Environmental Sciences, University of Exeter, Exeter, UK

Abstract

Several recent studies indicate that supplementation of the diet with inorganic nitrate results in a significant reduction in pulmonary O_2 uptake during sub-maximal exercise, an effect that appears to be related to enhanced skeletal muscle efficiency. The physiological mechanisms responsible for this effect are not completely understood but are presumably linked to the bioconversion of ingested nitrate into nitrite and thence to nitric oxide. Nitrite and/or nitric oxide may influence muscle contractile efficiency perhaps via effects on sarcoplasmic reticulum calcium handling or actin-myosin interaction, and may also improve the efficiency of mitochondrial oxidative phosphorylation. A reduced O_2 cost of exercise can be observed within 3 h of the consumption of 5–6 mmol of nitrate, and this effect can be preserved for at least 15 days provided that the same 'dose' of nitrate is consumed daily. A reduced O_2 cost of exercise following nitrate supplementation has now been reported for several types of exercise including cycling, walking, running, and knee extension exercise. Dietary nitrate supplementation has been reported to extend the time to exhaustion during high-intensity constant work rate exercise by 16–25% and to enhance cycling performance over 4, 10, and 16.1 km by 1–2% in recreationally active and moderately trained subjects. Although nitrate appears to be a promising 'new' ergogenic aid, additional research is required to determine the scope of its effects in different populations and different types of exercise.
Copyright © 2013 Nestec Ltd., Vevey/S. Karger AG, Basel

The Nitrate-Nitrite-Nitric Oxide Pathway

Nitric oxide (NO) is an important physiological signaling molecule that can modulate skeletal muscle function through its role in the regulation of blood flow, contractility, glucose and calcium homeostasis, and mitochondrial respi-

Table 1. Nitrate content (mg/100 g fresh weight) of selected vegetables

Nitrate content	Vegetable
Very high (>250)	beetroot, spinach, lettuce, rocket, celery, cress, chervil
High (100–250)	celeriac, fennel, leek, endive, parsley
Medium (50–100)	cabbage, savoy cabbage, turnip, dill
Low (20–50)	broccoli, carrot, cauliflower, cucumber, pumpkin
Very low (<20)	asparagus, aubergine, onion, mushroom, pea, pepper, potato, sweet potato, tomato

ration and biogenesis [1]. Until quite recently, it was considered that NO was generated solely through the oxidation of the amino acid L-arginine in a reaction catalyzed by NO synthase (NOS), and that nitrite (NO_2^-) and nitrate (NO_3^-) were inert by-products of this process [2]. However, it is now clear that these metabolites can be recycled back into bioactive NO under certain physiological conditions [3, 4]. The reduction of NO_3^- to NO_2^- and subsequently of NO_2^- to NO may be important as a means to increase NO production when NO synthesis by the NOS enzymes is impaired [5] and in conditions of low oxygen availability, as may occur in skeletal muscle during exercise.

In addition to being created through the NOS-catalyzed production of NO from L-arginine, tissue concentrations of NO_3^- and NO_2^- can be increased by dietary means. Vegetables account for 60–80% of the daily NO_3^- intake in a Western diet [6] with green leafy vegetables such as lettuce, spinach and beetroot being particularly rich in NO_3^- [7] (table 1). Ingested inorganic NO_3^- is rapidly absorbed from the gut and passes into the systemic circulation with peak plasma [NO_3^-] being observed approximately 60 min after ingestion [4]. While some 60% of the systemic NO_3^- is excreted in the urine [4]), 25% passes into the enterosalivary circulation and becomes highly concentrated in the saliva [8]. In the mouth, facultative anaerobic bacteria on the surface of the tongue reduce NO_3^- to NO_2^- [9]. This NO_2^- is swallowed and reduced to NO and other reactive nitrogen intermediates within the acidic environment of the stomach [10, 11]. However, some NO_2^- is absorbed to increase circulating plasma [NO_2^-] with the peak concentration being attained 2–3 h following NO_3^- ingestion [8, 12]. Therefore, dietary NO_3^- supplementation represents a practical method to increase circulating plasma [NO_2^-] and thus NO bioavailability. This has been demonstrated after ingestion of sodium nitrate ($NaNO_3$) [8 and 13–15], potassium nitrate [16], as well as NO_3^--rich beetroot juice [17–22]. Interestingly, the characteristic rise in plasma [NO_2^-] following an oral NO_3^- bolus is largely abolished by the use of antibacterial mouthwash [23], indicating that the reduction of NO_3^- to NO_2^- in humans is critically dependent on the oral bacterial NO_3^- reductases.

The final step in the NO_3^--NO_2^--NO pathway is the one electron reduction of NO_2^- to NO. This reaction is potentiated in hypoxic [24] and acidic [25] environments such as those which may exist in skeletal muscle during exercise [26]. The existence of an alternative NO generation pathway is important as it promotes NO synthesis under conditions that would otherwise limit the production of NO from NOS, ensuring that NO synthesis can occur across a wide range of cellular O_2 tensions. It is important to note, however, that NO_2^- may itself induce physiological effects independent of its reduction to NO [27].

The purpose of this paper is to provide a brief review of the available literature which supports a role for dietary nitrate supplementation in enhancing exercise performance in healthy humans. Given the importance of NO in vascular and metabolic control, there are sound theoretical reasons why augmenting NO bioavailability might be important in optimizing skeletal muscle function during exercise. Recent evidence indicates that elevating plasma $[NO_2^-]$ through dietary nitrate supplementation is associated with enhanced muscle efficiency, fatigue resistance and performance. The mechanistic bases for this effect are considered and practical recommendations for nitrate supplementation by athletes are provided.

Nitrate and Exercise

In 2007, Larsen et al. [15] reported that 3 days of $NaNO_3$ supplementation increased plasma $[NO_2^-]$ and reduced the O_2 cost of sub-maximal cycle exercise. Blood [lactate], heart rate and minute ventilation ($\dot{V}_E$) were not significantly altered. These findings were highly surprising because it is well established that the O_2 cost of exercising at a given sub-maximal power output is essentially 'fixed'. For example, during cycle ergometry, it is expected that pulmonary O_2 uptake ($\dot{V}_{O_2}$) will increase by approximately 10 ml per minute for every additional watt of external power output. The efficiency of exercise is considered to be independent of age, health status and physical fitness and, prior to the study of Larsen et al. [15], had been reported to be essentially unaffected by a variety of acute or chronic interventions [28]. Long-term endurance training may elicit some improvements in exercise efficiency, and it is known that efficiency is an important determinant of endurance exercise performance [29]. The results of Larsen et al. [15] were therefore exciting because they suggested that a short-term dietary intervention might improve exercise efficiency and have the potential to enhance performance.

The initial findings of Larsen et al. [15] were corroborated in the study of Bailey et al. [17] in which NO_3^- was administered in the form of beetroot juice.

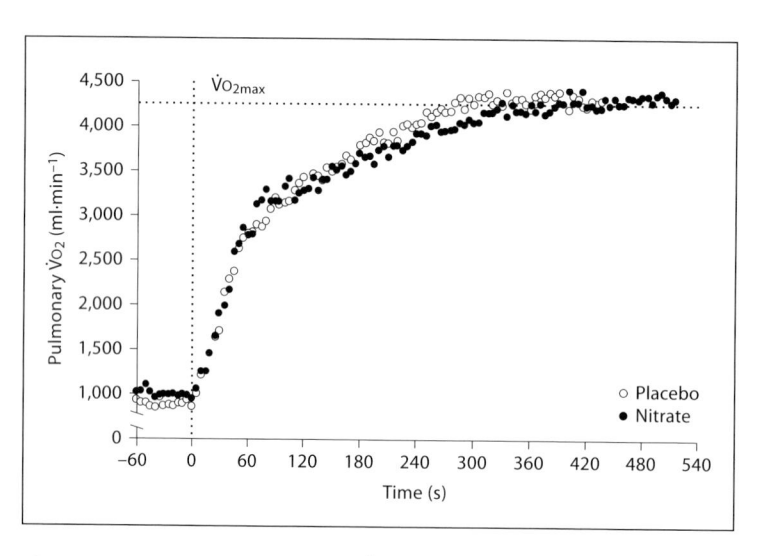

Fig. 1. Pulmonary oxygen uptake ($\dot{V}_{O_2}$) for a representative individual during severe-intensity cycle exercise continued until the limit of tolerance following nitrate (beetroot juice) and placebo supplementation. The dotted vertical line represents the abrupt imposition of the work rate from a baseline of 'unloaded' cycling. The dotted horizontal line represents the $\dot{V}_{O_2max}$ of the representative individual. Note the reduced $\dot{V}_{O_2}$ 'slow component', delayed attainment of the $\dot{V}_{O_2max}$ and longer time to exhaustion following nitrate supplementation.

Following 3 days of beetroot juice supplementation, the plasma [NO_2^-] was doubled, the steady-state $\dot{V}_{O_2}$ during moderate-intensity exercise was reduced, and the $\dot{V}_{O_2}$ 'slow component' during severe-intensity exercise was attenuated (fig. 1). As highlighted above, it is striking that a short-term, natural dietary intervention can improve the efficiency of muscular work.

The reduction in steady-state $\dot{V}_{O_2}$ after NO_3^- supplementation was of the order of 5% in the studies of Larsen et al. [15] and Bailey et al. [17] in which supplementation was continued for 3–6 days. A similar reduction in steady-state $\dot{V}_{O_2}$ during moderate-intensity cycle ergometry has been reported following acute NO_3^- treatment: 60 min following $NaNO_3$ administration [14] and 2.5 h following beetroot juice ingestion [21]. The improved exercise efficiency was sustained when NO_3^- supplementation was continued for 15 days [21] (fig. 2). This indicates that longer term NO_3^- supplementation does not elicit greater improvements in exercise efficiency but also, importantly, that tolerance to the intervention does not develop (at least up to 15 days). The reduction in $\dot{V}_{O_2}$ following NO_3^- administration is not unique to cycling exercise, having also been observed during two-legged knee-extensor exercise [16] and treadmill walking and running [19]. Importantly, no reduction in $\dot{V}_{O_2}$ was observed compared to a control

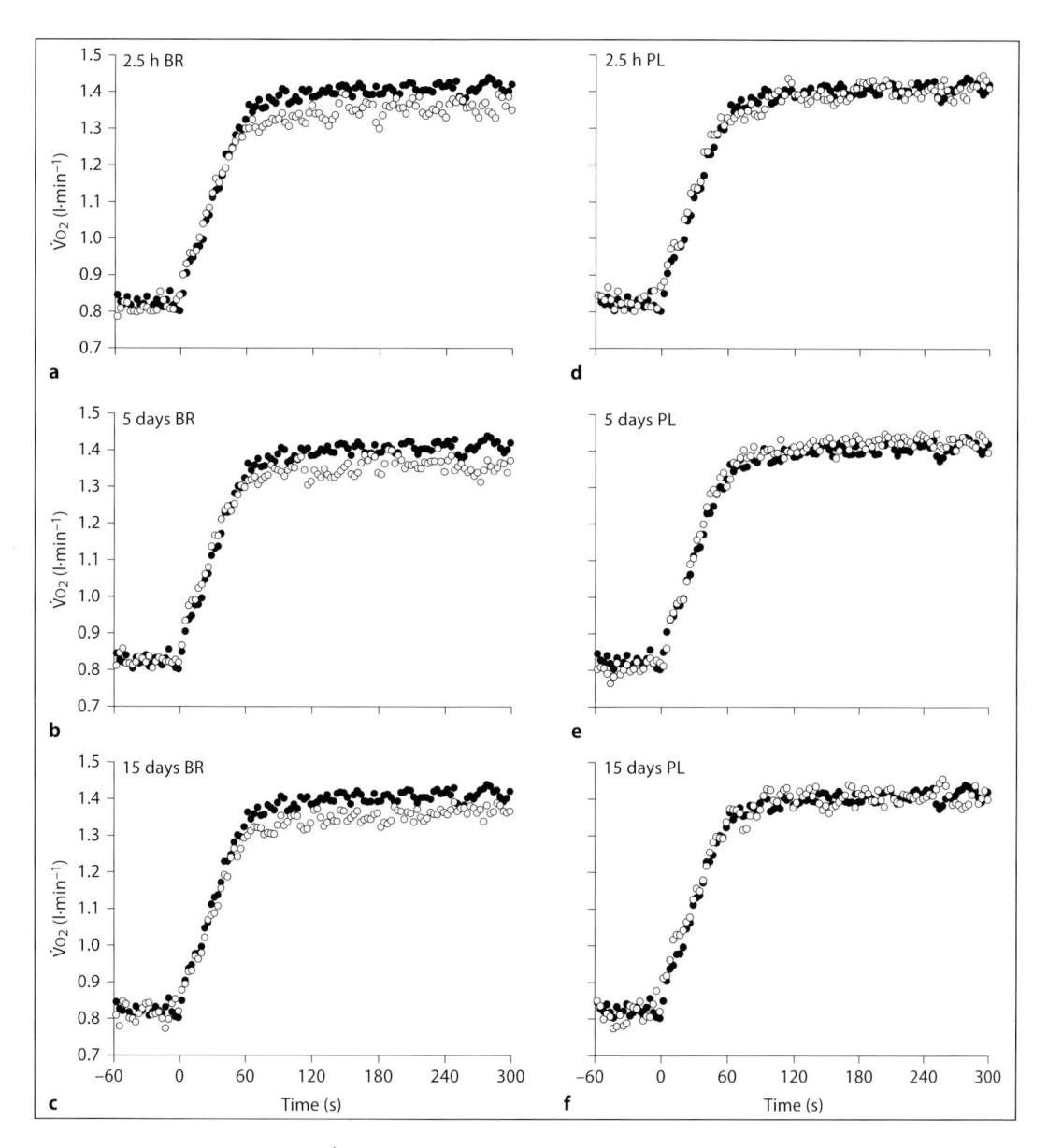

Fig. 2. The group mean $\dot{V}_{O_2}$ profiles during moderate-intensity exercise across 15-day supplementation periods with beetroot juice (BR) and placebo (PL) in comparison to pre-supplementation baseline (filled circles). Open circles indicate BR-supplemented trials in **a–c** and PL-supplemented trials in **d–f**. Error bars are omitted for clarity.

condition when the subjects were supplemented with a placebo beetroot juice that had been depleted of NO_3^- using an ion-exchange resin [19]. This confirms that NO_3^- is the key 'active' ingredient responsible for the physiological changes observed following beetroot juice supplementation. It does not rule out, however, a synergistic role for other components of beetroot juice such as antioxidants and polyphenols, which may facilitate the reduction of NO_3^- to NO_2^- and NO [30, 31]. Collectively, these results indicate that the reduced $\dot{V}_{O_2}$ following NO_3^- supplementation is reproducible and can be observed across a range of different supplementation regimens and exercise modalities.

Exercise Performance

Plasma $[NO_2^-]$ has recently been identified as an important correlate of exercise tolerance in healthy humans [32, 33]. Given that NO_3^- supplementation increases plasma $[NO_2^-]$, this intervention may therefore have the potential to improve exercise tolerance. This hypothesis was tested in the study of Bailey et al. [17]. Plasma $[NO_2^-]$ was doubled and exercise tolerance was enhanced by 16% following NO_3^--rich beetroot juice supplementation, suggesting that NO_3^- supplementation may indeed be ergogenic. Subsequent experiments have reported improvements in exercise tolerance of 25% during two-legged knee-extensor exercise [18], and of 15% during treadmill running [19] following 6 days of beetroot juice supplementation. Improved incremental exercise performance has also been noted following 6 days of beetroot juice supplementation during single-legged knee extension exercise [19] and after 15 days of beetroot juice supplementation during cycle exercise [21]. A trend for an improved exercise tolerance (+7%) during combined incremental arm and leg exercise was reported following 2 days of $NaNO_3$ supplementation [14]. This observation was made in concert with a reduced $\dot{V}_{O_2max}$ (–3%) which indicated that the subjects were more efficient even at maximal exertion following NO_3^- supplementation [14]. Incremental exercise performance was not significantly different (+2%) in trained athletes following acute $NaNO_3$ administration, despite a 4% statistically significant reduction in $\dot{V}_{O_2max}$ [34]. It is important to note that a reduction in $\dot{V}_{O_2max}$ is not always observed following NO_3^- supplementation [17, 21]. It is possible that the influence of NO_3^- supplementation on $\dot{V}_{O_2max}$ may be dependent on the exercise modality and/or the training status of the subjects.

It is well documented that exercise performance is compromised in hypoxia relative to normoxia. In this regard, it is noteworthy that Vanhatalo et al. [35] recently reported that nitrate supplementation with beetroot juice restored muscle performance in hypoxia (14% inspired O_2; equivalent to 4,000 m altitude) to

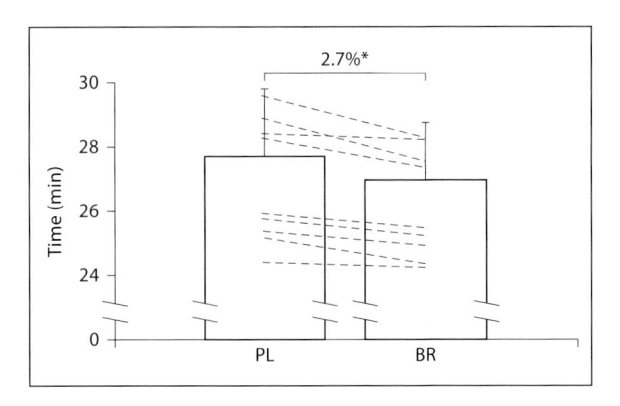

Fig. 3. Completion times for 16.1-km cycle time trial following BR and PL supplementation. The figure shows the group mean ± SEM completion times as columns and the dashed lines show the individual differences. * p < 0.01, completion time was significantly reduced following BR supplementation.

that observed in the normoxic control condition. Specifically, in hypoxia, nitrate supplementation resulted in a 20% extension of the time to exhaustion during high-intensity knee extensor exercise. Vanhatalo et al. [35] also reported that nitrate supplementation improved muscle oxidative function in hypoxia, suggesting that muscle oxygenation may have been enhanced. Consistent with this interpretation, Kenjale et al. [36] reported that beetroot juice supplementation resulted in a 17–18% longer time to claudication pain and peak walking time during incremental exercise in patients with peripheral arterial disease. The authors attributed the enhanced performance to NO_2^--related improvement in peripheral tissue oxygenation. Collectively, these results have potential performance implications for athletes competing at altitude and for improving functional capacity in clinical conditions where tissue O_2 supply may be compromised.

As summarized above, during constant work rate exercise, the improved exercise tolerance following NO_3^- supplementation has been reported to be in the range of 16–25% [17–19]. However, the magnitude of improvement in 'actual' exercise performance would be expected to be far smaller; indeed, using the predictions of Hopkins et al. [37], a ~20% improvement in time to exhaustion would be expected to correspond to an improvement in exercise performance (time taken to cover a set distance) of 1–2%. This hypothesis was tested in the study of Lansley et al. [20], where competitive but sub-elite cyclists completed, on separate days, 4.0- and 16.1-km time trials following acute beetroot juice ingestion. Consistent with the experimental hypothesis, NO_3^- administration improved 4.0- and 16.1-km time trial performance by ~2.7% compared to the placebo condition [20] (fig. 3). These improvements in exercise performance were consequent to the maintenance of a higher mean power output (+5–6%) and an increase in the power output/$\dot{V}_{O_2}$ ratio. Therefore, trained subjects were able to produce a higher power output for the same oxidative energy turnover (i.e. the inverse of a lower $\dot{V}_{O_2}$ for the same power output), resulting in an improved exercise performance following NO_3^- supplementation. The improved cycle time trial performance following nitrate supplementation reported by Lansley et al. [20] has recently been corroborated by Cermak et al. [38]. These authors reported that 6 days of beetroot juice supplementation (8 mmol/day) significantly reduced $\dot{V}_{O_2}$ at two sub-maximal work rates and improved mean power output and 10 km time trial performance (by 1.2%) in trained cyclists.

An improved exercise efficiency has been consistently reported when recreationally active humans ($\dot{V}_{O_2max}$ values typically between 45–55 ml·kg^{-1}·min^{-1}) have been supplemented with NO_3^- [13–15, 17–21]. However, Bescós et al. [34] recently reported that acute $NaNO_3$ ingestion did not significantly improve submaximal exercise efficiency in trained subjects ($\dot{V}_{O_2max}$ of 65 ml·kg^{-1}·min^{-1}). It is important to note that plasma [NO_2^-] was only increased by 16% in this study, whereas previous studies have observed far greater increases in plasma [NO_2^-] following NO_3^- supplementation, of as much as 100% [13–15, 17–21]. The resting plasma [NO_3^-] and [NO_2^-] is higher in athletes [39, 40], which may reduce the scope for NO_3^- supplementation to improve exercise efficiency in this population. Alternatively, more highly trained individuals may require a larger NO_3^- dose to elicit similar changes in plasma [NO_2^-] and exercise efficiency to those observed in recreationally active participants. It should also be considered that highly trained subjects are likely to have both higher NOS activity and greater mitochondrial and capillary density, which might limit the development of hypoxia and acidosis in skeletal muscle during exercise. Further research is needed to elucidate the influence of NO_3^- supplementation on exercise efficiency in athletes.

Mechanisms

The reduced O_2 cost of exercise following nitrate supplementation is not associated with an elevated blood [lactate] [15, 17], suggesting that there is no compensatory increase in anaerobic energy production as might be expected if oxidative metabolism were somehow inhibited. This indicates that nitrate supplementation results in a 'real' improvement in muscle efficiency. Theoretically, a lower O_2 cost of exercise for the same power output could result from: (1) a lower adenosine triphosphate (ATP) cost of muscle contraction for the same force production (i.e. improved muscle contractile efficiency), or (2) a lower O_2

consumption for the same rate of oxidative ATP resynthesis [i.e. improved metabolic (mitochondrial) efficiency].

Bailey et al. [18] investigated the first of these possibilities using calibrated ^{31}P-magnetic resonance spectroscopy. This procedure permitted the in vivo assessment of absolute muscle concentration changes in phosphocreatine ([PCr]), inorganic phosphate ([P$_i$]), and adenosine diphosphate ([ADP]), as well as pH. The ATP supply contributed by PCr hydrolysis, anaerobic glycolysis and oxidative phosphorylation during knee-extensor exercise was also calculated. The estimated ATP turnover rates from PCr hydrolysis and oxidative phosphorylation were lower following 6 days of beetroot juice supplementation, and contributed to a significant reduction in the estimated total ATP turnover rate during both low- and high-intensity exercise [18]. It is known that the ATP turnover rate in contracting myocytes is determined, in the large part, by the activity of actomyosin ATPase and Ca^{2+}-ATPase [41]. NO has been shown to slow myosin cycling kinetics [42] and to reduce Ca^{2+}-ATPase activity [43]. As such, elevated NO production following beetroot juice supplementation may have reduced skeletal muscle ATP turnover by reducing the activity of actomyosin ATPase and/or Ca^{2+}-ATPase. The intramuscular accumulation of ADP and P$_i$, and the extent of PCr depletion, were also blunted following NO$_3^-$ supplementation [18]. The smaller changes in [ADP], [P$_i$] and [PCr] following NO$_3^-$ supplementation would be predicted to reduce the stimuli for increasing oxidative phosphorylation [44, 45].

The accumulation of metabolites such as [ADP] and [P$_i$], and the rate of depletion of the finite intramuscular [PCr] reserves, are important contributors to muscle fatigue development [46, 47]. While the intramuscular [ADP], [P$_i$] and [PCr] were similar at exhaustion in the NO$_3^-$ and placebo conditions in the study of Bailey et al. [18] and also Vanhatalo et al. [35], the time taken to achieve these critical concentrations was delayed following NO$_3^-$ supplementation, and this, in part, may explain the improved exercise tolerance. In line with these data, dietary NO$_3^-$ supplementation has been shown to reduce the development of the $\dot{V}_{O_2}$ 'slow component' during high-intensity exercise such that the attainment of the $\dot{V}_{O_2max}$ is delayed and the tolerable duration of exercise is extended [17]. It should be noted that while the improved muscle efficiency and reduced metabolic perturbation may be responsible for the enhanced exercise tolerance observed following nitrate supplementation, it is possible that the intervention results in a simultaneous improvement in O$_2$ delivery to muscle loci that are most 'hypoxic' [35, 36]. If true, then this, too, might contribute to improved exercise performance.

The second possibility – that nitrate supplementation enhances mitochondrial efficiency – was recently examined by Larsen et al. [13]. These authors isolated mitochondria from the vastus lateralis muscle of healthy humans supplemented with NaNO$_3^-$. The resultant mitochondrial suspension was added to a reaction medium containing the substrates pyruvate and malate, allowing mitochondrial respiration to be investigated. With a submaximal rate of ADP infusion, the mitochondrial P/O ratio (the amount of ADP administered divided by O$_2$ consumed) was significantly increased [13]. The respiratory control ratio, which is the ratio between state 3 (coupled) and state 4 (uncoupled) respiration, was also significantly increased with NaNO$_3^-$ supplementation, as was the maximal rate of ATP production through oxidative phosphorylation. State 2 respiration, indicative of back leakage of protons through the inner mitochondrial membrane, and state 4 respiration were both reduced with NaNO$_3^-$ [13]. Therefore, these data indicated that NO$_3^-$ supplementation reduced proton leakage and uncoupled respiration, which increased the mitochondrial P/O ratio. The increased P/O ratio following NO$_3^-$ supplementation was correlated with the reduction in whole body O$_2$ during exercise [13]. Taken together with the findings of Bailey et al. [18], it appears that NO$_3^-$ supplementation may improve exercise efficiency by improving the efficiency of both muscle contraction (reduced ATP cost of force production) and mitochondrial oxidative phosphorylation (increased P/O ratio).

Practical Recommendations

The available evidence indicates that dietary supplementation with 5–7 mmol nitrate (approximately 0.1 mmol/kg body mass) results in a significant increase in plasma [nitrite] and associated physiological effects including a lower resting blood pressure, reduced pulmonary O$_2$ uptake during sub-maximal exercise and enhanced exercise tolerance or performance [13–15, 17–21, 35, 36, 38]. This 'dose' of nitrate can readily be achieved through the consumption of 0.5 l of beetroot juice (or an equivalent high-nitrate foodstuff). Following a 5- to 6-mmol 'bolus' of nitrate, plasma [nitrite] typically peaks within 2–3 h and remains elevated for a further 6–9 h before declining towards baseline [22]. Therefore, it is recommended that nitrate is consumed approximately 3 h prior to competition or training. A daily dose of a high-nitrate supplement is required if plasma [nitrite] is to remain elevated.

Although nitrate supplementation appears to hold promise as an ergogenic aid, it is important to recognize that there is still much that we do not know. Firstly, most of the published studies to date have involved recreational or moderately trained subjects, and it is not known if nitrate supplementation substantially elevates plasma [NO$_2^-$] or is ergogenic in elite athletes. Secondly, while the ingestion of 5–6 mmol of nitrate appears to be effective, studies are ongoing to determine the 'dose-response' relationship between nitrate supplementation and changes in exercise efficiency and performance; this will shed light on the 'optimal' loading regimen for performance enhancement. Thirdly, while nitrate supplementation appears to be ergogenic in continuous maximal activity of 5–25 min duration, possible effects on short-term high-intensity exercise, intermittent exercise, and long-term endurance exercise performance have not been investigated. Finally, it is presently unclear if, and in what ways, sustained dietary nitrate supplementation might impact upon adaptations to training: on the one hand, increased NO bioavailability might simulate mitochondrial biogenesis and angiogenesis; on the other hand, nitrate has anti-oxidant properties that might blunt cellular adaptations.

It is important to note that dietary or environmental exposure to NO_3^- has historically been considered to be harmful to human health due to a possible increased risk of gastric cancer [48]. More recent evidence challenges this view and indicates that NO_3^- ingestion (at least through dietary means) may instead confer benefits to health [49, 50]. Until more is known, it is recommended that athletes wishing to explore possible ergogenic effects of nitrate supplementation employ a natural, rather than pharmacological, approach [51].

Disclosure Statement

The author declares that no financial or other conflict of interest exists in relation to the content of the chapter.

References

1 Stamler JS, Meissner G: Physiology of nitric oxide in skeletal muscle. Physiol Rev 2001; 81:209–237.
2 Moncada S, Higgs A: The L-arginine-nitric oxide pathway. N Engl J Med 1993;329: 2002–2012.
3 Bryan NS: Nitrite in nitric oxide biology: cause or consequence? A systems-based review. Free Radic Biol Med 2006;41:691–701.
4 Lundberg JO, Weitzberg E: NO generation from inorganic nitrate and nitrite: role in physiology, nutrition and therapeutics. Arch Pharm Res 2009;32:1119–1126.
5 Bryan NS, Calvert JW, Gundewar S, Lefer DJ: Dietary nitrite restores NO homeostasis and is cardioprotective in endothelial nitric oxide synthase-deficient mice. Free Radic Biol Med 2008;45:468–474.
6 Ysart G, Miller P, Barrett G, et al: Dietary exposures to nitrate in the UK. Food Addit Contam 1999;16:521–532.
7 Bryan NS, Hord NG: Dietary nitrates and nitrites: the physiological context for potential health benefits; in Bryan NS (ed): Food, Nutrition and the Nitric Oxide Pathway. Pennsylvania, DEStech Publications, 2010, pp 59–78.

8 Lundberg JO, Govoni M: Inorganic nitrate is a possible source for systemic generation of nitric oxide. Free Radic Biol Med 2004;37: 395–400.
9 Duncan C, Dougall H, Johnston P, et al: Chemical generation of nitric oxide in the mouth from the enterosalivary circulation of dietary nitrate. Nat Med 1995;1:546–551.
10 Benjamin N, O'Driscoll F, Dougall H, et al: Stomach NO synthesis. Nature 1994;368: 502–503.
11 Lundberg JO, Weitzberg E, Cole JA, Benjamin N: Nitrate, bacteria and human health. Nat Rev Microbiol 2004;2:593–602.
12 Dejam A, Hunter CJ, Schechter AN, Gladwin MT: Emerging role of nitrite in human biology. Blood Cells Mol Dis 2004;32:423–429.
13 Larsen FJ, Schiffer TA, Borniquel S, et al: Dietary inorganic nitrate improves mitochondrial efficiency in humans. Cell Metab 2011;13:149–159.
14 Larsen FJ, Weitzberg E, Lundberg JO, Ekblom B: Dietary nitrate reduces maximal oxygen consumption while maintaining work performance in maximal exercise. Free Radic Biol Med 2010;48:342–347.
15 Larsen FJ, Weitzberg E, Lundberg JO, Ekblom B: Effects of dietary nitrate on oxygen cost during exercise. Acta Physiol 2007;191: 59–66.
16 Kapil V, Milsom AB, Okorie M, et al: Inorganic nitrate supplementation lowers blood pressure in humans: role for nitrite-derived NO. Hypertension 2010;56:274–281.
17 Bailey SJ, Winyard P, Vanhatalo A, et al: Dietary nitrate supplementation reduces the O_2 cost of low-intensity exercise and enhances tolerance to high-intensity exercise in humans. J Appl Physiol 2009;107:1144–1155.
18 Bailey SJ, Fulford J, Vanhatalo A, et al: Dietary nitrate supplementation enhances muscle contractile efficiency during knee-extensor exercise in humans. J Appl Physiol 2010;109:135–148.
19 Lansley KE, Winyard PG, Fulford J, et al: Dietary nitrate supplementation reduces the O_2 cost of walking and running: a placebo-controlled study. J Appl Physiol 2011;110: 591–600.
20 Lansley KE, Winyard PG, Bailey SJ, et al: Acute dietary nitrate supplementation improves cycling time trial performance. Med Sci Sports Exerc 2011;43:1125–1131.
21 Vanhatalo A, Bailey SJ, Blackwell JR, et al: Acute and chronic effects of dietary nitrate supplementation on blood pressure and the physiological responses to moderate-intensity and incremental exercise. Am J Physiol Regul Integr Comp Physiol 2010;299:R1121–R1131.
22 Webb AJ, Patel N, Loukogeorgakis S, et al: Acute blood pressure lowering, vasoprotective, and antiplatelet properties of dietary nitrate via bioconversion to nitrite. Hypertension 2008;51:784–790.
23 Govoni M, Jansson EA, Weitzberg E, Lundberg JO: The increase in plasma nitrite after a dietary nitrate load is markedly attenuated by an antibacterial mouthwash. Nitric Oxide 2008;19:333–337.
24 Castello PR, David PS, McClure T, et al: Mitochondrial cytochrome oxidase produces nitric oxide under hypoxic conditions: implications for oxygen sensing and hypoxic signaling in eukaryotes. Cell Metab 2006;3: 277–287.
25 Modin A, Björne H, Herulf M, et al: Nitrite-derived nitric oxide: a possible mediator of 'acidic-metabolic' vasodilation. Acta Physiol Scand 2001;171:9–16.
26 Richardson RS, Leigh JS, Wagner PD, Noyszewski EA: Cellular PO_2 as a determinant of maximal mitochondrial O_2 consumption in trained human skeletal muscle. J Appl Physiol 1999;87:325–331.
27 Bryan NS, Fernandez BO, Bauer SM, et al: Nitrite is a signaling molecule and regulator of gene expression in mammalian tissues. Nat Chem Biol 2005;1:290–297.
28 Jones AM, Poole DC: Introduction to oxygen uptake kinetics and historical development of the discipline; in Jones AM, Poole DC (eds): Oxygen Uptake Kinetics in Sport, Exercise and Medicine. London, Routledge, 2005, pp 3–35.
29 Jones AM, Carter H: The effect of endurance training on parameters of aerobic fitness. Sports Med 2000;29:373–386.
30 Carlsson S, Wiklund NP, Engstrand L, et al: Effects of pH, nitrite, and ascorbic acid on nonenzymatic nitric oxide generation and bacterial growth in urine. Nitric Oxide 2001; 5:580–586.
31 Gago B, Lundberg JO, Barbosa RM, Laranjinha J: Red wine-dependent reduction of nitrite to nitric oxide in the stomach. Free Radic Biol Med 2007;43:1233–1242.

32 Rassaf T, Lauer T, Heiss C, et al: Nitric oxide synthase-derived plasma nitrite predicts exercise capacity. Br J Sports Med 2007;41:669–673.

33 Dreissigacker U, Wendt M, Wittke T, et al: Positive correlation between plasma nitrite and performance during high-intensive exercise but not oxidative stress in healthy men. Nitric Oxide 2010;23:128–135.

34 Bescós R, Rodríguez FA, Iglesias X, et al: Acute administration of inorganic nitrate reduces O_{2peak} in endurance athletes. Med Sci Sports Exerc 2011;43:1979–1986.

35 Vanhatalo A, Fulford J, Bailey SJ, et al: Dietary nitrate reduces muscle metabolic perturbation and improves exercise tolerance in hypoxia. J Physiol 2011;589:5517–5528.

36 Kenjale AA, Ham KL, Stabler T, et al: Dietary nitrate supplementation enhances exercise performance in peripheral arterial disease. J Appl Physiol 2011;110:1582–1591.

37 Hopkins WG, Hawley JA, Burke LM: Design and analysis of research on sport performance enhancement. Med Sci Sports Exerc 1999;31:472–485.

38 Cermak NM, Gibala MJ, van Loon LJC: Nitrate supplementation's improvement of 10-km time-trial performance in trained cyclists. Int J Sport Nutr Exerc Metab 2012;22:64–71.

39 Jungersten L, Ambring A, Wall B, Wennmalm A: Both physical fitness and acute exercise regulate nitric oxide formation in healthy humans. J Appl Physiol 1997;82:760–764.

40 Schena F, Cuzzolin L, Rossi L, et al: Plasma nitrite/nitrate and erythropoietin levels in cross-country skiers during altitude training. J Sports Med Phys Fit 2002;42:129–134.

41 Barclay CJ, Woledge RC, Curtin NA: Energy turnover for Ca^{2+} cycling in skeletal muscle. J Muscle Res Cell Mot 2007;28:259–274.

42 Evangelista AM, Rao VS, Filo AR, et al: Direct regulation of striated muscle myosins by nitric oxide and endogenous nitrosothiols. PLoS One 2010;5:e11209.

43 Ishii T, Sunami O, Saitoh N, et al: Inhibition of skeletal muscle sarcoplasmic reticulum Ca^{2+}-ATPase by nitric oxide. FEBS Lett 1998;440:218–222.

44 Chance B, Williams GR: Respiratory enzymes in oxidative phosphorylation. I. Kinetics of oxygen utilization. J Biol Chem 1955;217:383–393.

45 Mahler M: First-order kinetics of muscle oxygen consumption, and equivalent proportionality between QO_2 and phosphorylcreatine level. Implications for the control of respiration. J Gen Physiol 1985;86:135–165.

46 Allen DG, Lamb GD, Westerblad H: Skeletal muscle fatigue: cellular mechanisms. Physiol Rev 2008;88:287–332.

47 Jones AM, Wilkerson DP, DiMenna F, et al: Muscle metabolic responses to exercise above and below the 'critical power' assessed using ^{31}P-MRS. Am J Physiol Regul Integr Comp Physiol 2008;294:585–593.

48 Tannenbaum SR, Weisman M, Fett D: The effect of nitrate intake on nitrite formation in human saliva. Food Cosmet Toxicol 1976;14:549–552.

49 Bryan NS, Hord NG: Regulations gone awry: Addressing public health concerns; in Bryan NS (ed): Food, Nutrition and the Nitric Oxide Pathway. Pennsylvania, DEStech Publications, 2010, pp 153–166.

50 Gilchrist M, Winyard PG, Benjamin N: Dietary nitrate – good or bad? Nitric Oxide 2010;22:104–109.

51 Lundberg JO, Larsen FJ, Weitzberg E: Supplementation with nitrate and nitrite salts in exercise: a word of caution. J Appl Physiol 2011;111:616–617.

Questions and Answers

Question 1: Beetroot supplementation has some unwanted side effects: what are they?

Answer: Well, it can stain the body fluids and give the urine, saliva, and stool a pink/red/purple color. It is not really an unwanted or harmful side effect, but you just need to be aware that it is going to change color of certain excretions.

That said, at least you know then that it has been effective in actually being absorbed into your body.

Question 2: Could you explain the mechanism by which nitrate can improve performance?

Answer: Yes, we think that when the nitrate is taken through a foodstuff initially it gets converted into nitrite in the body. So, the nitrate is swallowed and then transported into the enterosalivary circulation, and it reenters the mouth in the saliva where the bacteria in the mouth reduce the nitrate to nitrite. The nitrite is subsequently swallowed and then can be absorbed into the bloodstream. So, the plasma nitrite concentration is increased following beetroot juice or other forms of dietary nitrate supplementation. The nitrite is then transported in the blood and can be broken down further into nitric oxide in areas where it is most needed. We think that this is important in performance terms because nitric oxide has been shown to regulate muscle blood flow and also to regulate muscle contraction energetics and possibly mitochondrial efficiency as well. So, there are a number of reasons by which nitrate (as long as it is turned into nitric oxide) could be useful to physiological function and to exercise performance.

Question 3: What is your practical recommendation for beetroot juice supplementation in athletes?

Answer: We are still experimenting with the appropriate dose in order to get the maximum response. The studies that we have done so far involve the consumption of around 6 mmol nitrate. That is contained in about a half a liter of normal beetroot juice, although that can vary from company to company. It is possible now to buy beetroot juice shots which are a concentrated form of beetroot juice which contains the same amount of nitrate but in a reduced volume of fluid. An important thing is that the nitrate is consumed about 2 or 3 h before exercise is commenced, because that gives sufficient time for the nitrate to be converted into nitrite.

Question 4: Should athletes consume it over a long or a short time period?

Answer: That is another very good question. We do not know the answer to that question right know. We know there is an acute effect. If you take nitrate in the diet, then 2 or 3 h later your blood pressure will be a bit lower; if you exercise, your oxygen uptake will also be slightly lower, and your performance may be slightly improved. And we can continue to supplement for up to 15 days, which is as far as we have gone in our studies, and we do not lose that effectiveness. But, that said, we do not know whether continued nitrate supplementation may or may not enhance adaptations to training.

Nutritional Strategies to Support Adaptation to High-Intensity Interval Training in Team Sports

Martin J. Gibala

McMaster University, Hamilton, Ont., Canada

Abstract

Team sports are characterized by intermittent high-intensity activity patterns. Typically, play consists of short periods of very intense or all-out efforts interspersed with longer periods of low-intensity activity. Fatigue is a complex, multi-factorial process, but intense intermittent exercise performance can potentially be limited by reduced availability of substrates stored in skeletal muscle and/or metabolic by-products associated with fuel breakdown. High-intensity interval training (HIT) has been shown to induce adaptations in skeletal muscle that enhance the capacity for both oxidative and non-oxidative metabolism. Nutrient availability is a potent modulator of many acute physiological responses to exercise, including various molecular signaling pathways that are believed to regulate cellular adaptation to training. Several nutritional strategies have also been reported to acutely alter metabolism and enhance intermittent high-intensity exercise performance. However, relatively little is known regarding the effect of chronic interventions, and whether supplementation over a period of weeks or months augments HIT-induced physiological remodeling and promotes greater performance adaptations. Theoretically, a nutritional intervention could augment HIT adaptation by improving energy metabolism during exercise, which could facilitate greater total work and an enhanced chronic training stimulus, or promoting some aspect of the adaptive response during recovery, which could lead to enhanced physiological adaptations over time.

Copyright © 2013 Nestec Ltd., Vevey/S. Karger AG, Basel

Introduction

Team sports are characterized by intermittent high-intensity activity patterns. For a given player, the metabolic demands will vary depending on many factors including position, playing style and game strategy. Typically however, play consists of short periods of very intense or all-out efforts interspersed with longer periods of low-intensity activity, and training programs are at least partly designed to simulate this activity pattern. Much of our knowledge regarding the metabolic demands of training and competition in team sport comes from studies conducted on soccer players [1]. For example, top players can perform 150–250 brief intense sprints over 10–15 m while covering a total of 10–12 km during the course of a match. The intermittent nature of this type of activity requires a high capacity for both aerobic (oxidative) and anaerobic (non-oxidative) energy provision, with skeletal muscle glycogen being a predominant fuel source [2].

Metabolic Factors Limiting Performance during Intense Intermittent Exercise

Fatigue is a complex, multi-factorial process, but intense intermittent exercise performance can potentially be limited by reduced availability of substrates stored in skeletal muscle (e.g. glycogen) and/or metabolic by-products associated with fuel breakdown [3]. Almost half the individual muscle fibers examined after a standard soccer match were either completely or nearly completely emptied of glycogen, suggesting that fiber-specific depletion may have impaired force-generating capacity and contributed to the reduced sprint performance observed after the second half of play [2]. Another potential mechanism related to glycogen metabolism is the metabolic acidosis that can occur during intense muscle contraction, owing to increased hydrogen ion accumulation in conjunction with lactate production. Intense intermittent exercise can cause significant decreases in muscle pH that are associated with impaired metabolic and contractile processes [3], although the acute change in muscle pH reported after a soccer game was modest and unrelated to the decline in sprint performance observed [2]. Nonetheless, a high buffering capacity has been associated with enhanced high-intensity exercise performance [4].

Skeletal Muscle Adaptation to High-Intensity Interval Training

High-intensity interval training (HIT) is infinitely variable, and the specific physiological adaptations induced by this form of training are determined by numerous factors including the precise nature of the exercise stimulus, i.e. the intensity, duration and number of intervals performed as well as the nature and duration of the recovery periods [5]. Interval intensity is a critical variable that

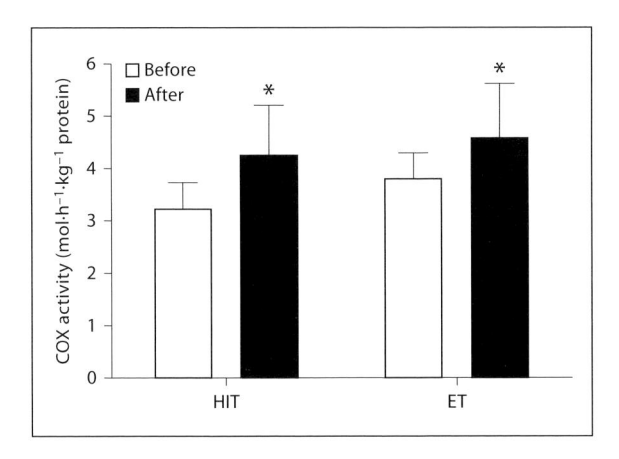

Fig. 1. Maximal activity of cytochrome oxidase (COX) measured in resting muscle biopsy samples obtained before and after 6 sessions of HIT or endurance training (ET) over 2 weeks. * $p \leq 0.05$ versus pre-training (main effect for time). Redrawn from Gibala and McGee [6] with permission.

can be quantified in various ways, but HIT generally refers to repeated efforts that correspond to ≥90% of maximal heart rate or ≥85% of peak oxygen uptake (VO_{2peak}). Numerous short-term HIT protocols – mainly cycling or running models – have been shown to induce adaptations in skeletal muscle that enhance the capacity for both oxidative and non-oxidative metabolism [6–9]. As little as sessions of HIT over 2 weeks can increase the content of mitochondrial enzymes (fig. 1), alter substrate metabolism (such that muscle glycogen is used more 'efficiently' during exercise), and improve buffering capacity [6, 7]. Much of this work has been conducted on recreational athletes, and while short-term HIT can also improve performance in high-trained subjects, the precise mechanisms responsible are less clear [9]. It has been suggested that training-induced changes in Na^+/K^+ pump activity may help to preserve cell excitability and force production, thereby delay fatigue development during intense exercise [8].

Recent data suggest that very intense HIT protocols may indeed provide a sufficient stimulus for mitochondrial adaptation in trained individuals. Psilander et al. [10] reported that a single bout of low-volume HIT (7 × 30-second all-out efforts) stimulated increases in mitochondrial gene expression that were comparable to or greater than the changes after more prolonged efforts (3 × 20-min bouts at ~87% of VO_{2peak}) in well-trained cyclists. Notably, of the two interventions, only the 30-second protocol stimulated an increase in mitochondrial transcription factor A, the downstream target of peroxisome-proliferator activated receptor-γ coactivator-1α, which is regarded as the master regulator of mitochondrial biogenesis in muscle [11]. The authors concluded that brief 'supramaximal' type interval training might be a time-efficient strategy to promote skeletal muscle adaptation in highly trained individuals. In this regard, Laursen [12] proposed that a polarized approach to training, in which ~75% of total training volume be performed at low intensities, with 10–15% performed at supra-maximal intensities may be the optimal training intensity distribution for elite athletes who compete in intense endurance events.

Potential Nutritional Strategies to Alter HIT Adaptation

Guidelines are available regarding the appropriate selection of food and fluids, timing of intake, and supplement choices [13], including recommendations by sports nutrition experts specifically tailored to team sport players [14, 15] and those who engage in power sports [16]. The general consensus is that athletes should consume a high-carbohydrate diet (6–12 g/kg per day) in order to maximize muscle glycogen availability and meet the energy demands of training and competition. However, there is also evidence to suggest that periodic training with reduced carbohydrate availability may augment HIT-induced adaptations in skeletal muscle [17], including one study that applied the 'train low' theory to a team sport model. Morton et al. [18] studied three groups of recreationally active men who performed 6 weeks of high-intensity intermittent running. Two groups of subjects trained twice per day, 2 days per week, such that half of their training was performed in a glycogen-reduced state, whereas the third group trained once per day, 4 days per week, under conditions of high carbohydrate availability. One of the 'low' groups received a carbohydrate drink prior to the second training session, whereas the other group received a nonenergetic placebo. The most intriguing finding was that training under conditions of reduced carbohydrate availability (i.e. the low group without the carbohydrate drink) provided an enhanced stimulus for skeletal muscle adaptation, such that the increase in oxidative enzymes was superior compared to the two carbohydrate-supplemented conditions. However, the training-induced improvements in a high-intensity intermittent running test were similar among all three groups of subjects. Thus, while periodic training with reduced glycogen availability stimulated greater muscle adaptations, this did not translate into improved performance. In the current volume, Hawley [pp. 1–14] considers in greater detail the potential effects of manipulating carbohydrate availability on training adaptation and performance.

Nutrient availability is a potent modulator of many acute physiological responses to exercise, including various molecular signaling pathways that are believed to regulate cellular adaptation to training [19]. While most studies have focused on the response to traditional endurance or resistance exercise, several recent investigations have reported that dietary manipulation can alter the acute molecular signaling response to high-intensity exercise. Guerra et al. [20] examined AMP-activated protein kinase (AMPK) signaling after a 30-second all-out cycling effort (Wingate test), which was performed in an overnight fasted state or following ingestion of a 75 glucose drink. Glucose ingestion blunted peak AMPKα phosphorylation 30 min after exercise and generally altered the acute signaling response during recovery, possibly via changes in circulating insulin concentration. Cochran et al. [21] reported that when two sessions of interval exercise were performed on the same day separated by several hours of recovery, manipulating food intake after the first (morning) exercise session influenced the acute skeletal muscle signaling response to the second (afternoon) session. Specifically, exercise-induced phosphorylation of p38 mitogen-activated protein kinase was higher when subjects ingested a non-energetic placebo drink during recovery as compared to a glucose beverage. The results from these two studies suggest that restricting carbohydrate availability can augment some acute signaling responses linked to mitochondrial biogenesis, consistent with the 'train low' theory described above. In contrast, Coffey et al. [22] showed that nutrient provision enhanced molecular signaling pathways linked to muscle growth after repeated sprint exercise. Specifically, ingestion of a carbohydrate-protein supplement was associated with coordinated increases in phosphorylation of the Akt-mTOR-S6K-rpS6 anabolic signaling cascade and myofibrillar protein synthesis during recovery, whereas no effect was observed when exercise was undertaken in the fasted state. The practical implication of this work is that manipulating food availability in close temporal proximity to high-intensity exercise can modulate the acute adaptive response of skeletal muscle, but the chronic implications – if any – of these short-term transient effects remain to be elucidated.

Several nutritional supplements have also been shown to acutely alter metabolism and enhance intermittent high-intensity exercise performance [14–16]. However, relatively little is known regarding the effect of chronic interventions, and whether supplementation over a period of weeks or months augments HIT-induced physiological remodeling and promotes greater performance adaptations. Theoretically, a nutritional intervention could augment the adaptation to HIT by (1) improving energy metabolism during acute high-intensity exercise (e.g. enhancing mitochondrial function), which could facilitate greater total work and an enhanced chronic training stimulus; (2) promoting some aspect of the acute molecular response to exercise (e.g. by increasing gene expression in recovery), which could lead to enhanced physiological adaptations over time, or (3) some combination of these two factors. A theoretical model by

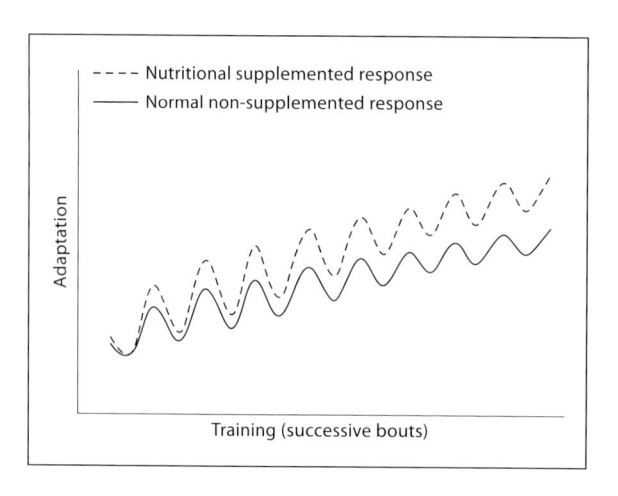

Fig. 2. Theoretical model by which nutritional manipulation could augment adaptation to HIT by 'optimizing' the effect of successive training bouts. While nutrient availability is a potent modulator of many acute responses to exercise, at present there is little direct evidence to support the model (i.e. in terms of specific physiological adaptations to HIT that are altered by chronic nutritional manipulation).

which nutritional manipulation could augment adaptation to HIT by 'optimizing' the effect of successive training bouts is shown in figure 2.

Limited evidence suggests that two supplements – sodium bicarbonate and β-alanine – could potentially augment training adaptations by altering muscle buffering capacity. Edge et al. [23] reported that subjects who ingested sodium bicarbonate over an 8-week high-intensity intermittent cycle training program, matched for total volume, experienced greater improvements in time-trial performance compared to a placebo group. Biopsies revealed no differences in several measured metabolites, but the authors posited the sodium bicarbonate group may have experienced greater gains in muscle oxidative capacity. A study conducted on rats showed that chronic bicarbonate ingestion in conjunction with HIT was associated with greater improvements in skeletal muscle mitochondrial mass and mitochondrial respiration, possibly due to reduced hydrogen ion accumulation during training [24]. The chapter by Burke in the current volume [pp. 15–26] reviews in greater detail the practice of bicarbonate loading to potentially improve performance during high-intensity exercise.

β-Alanine is a non-proteinogenic amino acid and rate-determining precursor (along with L-histidine) for the synthesis of carnosine, a dipeptide that functions as a physiologically relevant pH buffer in skeletal muscle [25]. β-Alanine supplementation is an effective means to increase muscle carnosine content, with daily doses of 4.8–6.4 g shown to increase muscle carnosine content by ~50–60% after 4 weeks [25]. Chronic β-alanine supplementation for up to 10 weeks has also been reported to improve acute high-intensity cycle exercise capacity [26] and augment resistance training-induced gains in strength [27]. However, no studies have directly investigated the potential for chronic β-alanine supplementation to alter skeletal muscle adaptations to HIT.

Conclusion

Several nutritional strategies have been shown to acutely alter metabolism and enhance intermittent high-intensity exercise performance, but little is known regarding the effect of chronic interventions. Nutritional compounds that alter muscle pH such as sodium bicarbonate and β-alanine are potential candidates, but training studies are warranted to determine whether supplementation over weeks or months augments HIT-induced physiological remodeling and/or promotes greater performance adaptations in humans.

Disclosure Statement

The author declares that no financial or other conflict of interest exists in relation to the content of the chapter.

References

1 Bangsbo J, Mohr M, Krustrup P: Physical and metabolic demands of training and match-play in the elite football player. J Sports Sci 2006;24:665–674.
2 Krustrup P, Mohr M, Steensberg A, et al: Muscle and blood metabolites during a soccer game: implications for sprint performance. Med Sci Sports Exerc 2006;38:1165–1174.
3 Girard O, Mendez-Villanueva A, Bishop D: Repeated-sprint ability. I. Factors contributing to fatigue. Sports Med 2011;41:673–694.
4 Sahlin K: Metabolic factors in fatigue. Sports Med 1992;13:99–107.
5 Laursen PB: Training for intense exercise performance: high-intensity or high-volume training? Scand J Med Sci Sports 2010; 20(suppl 2):1–10.
6 Gibala MJ, McGee SL: Metabolic adaptations to short-term high-intensity interval training: a little pain for a lot of gain? Exerc Sport Sci Rev 2008;36:58–63.
7 Gibala MJ, Little JP, van Essen M, et al: Short-term sprint interval versus traditional endurance training: similar initial adaptations in human skeletal muscle and exercise performance. J Physiol 2006;575:901–911.
8 Iaia FM, Bangsbo J: Speed endurance training is a powerful stimulus for physiological adaptations and performance improvements of athletes. Scand J Med Sci Sports 2010; 20(suppl 2):11–23.
9 Hawley JA, Myburgh KH, Noakes TD, Dennis SC: Training techniques to improve fatigue resistance and enhance endurance performance. J Sports Sci 1997;15:25–33.

10 Psilander N, Wang L, Westergren J, et al: Mitochondrial gene expression in elite cyclists: effects of high-intensity interval exercise. Eur J Appl Physiol 2010;110:597–606.
11 Olesen J, Kiilerich K, Pilegaard H: PGC-1alpha-mediated adaptations in skeletal muscle. Pflugers Arch 2010;460:153–162.
12 Laursen PB: Training for intense exercise performance: high-intensity or high-volume training? Scand J Med Sci Sports 2010; 20(suppl 2):1–10.
13 American Dietetic Association, Dietitians of Canada, American College of Sports Medicine: Nutrition and athletic performance. Med Sci Sports Exerc 2009;41:709–731.
14 Bishop D: Dietary supplements and team-sport performance. Sports Med 2010;40: 995–1017.
15 Mujika I, Burke LM: Nutrition in team sports. Ann Nutr Metab 2010;57(suppl 2):26–35.
16 Stellingwerff T, Maughan RJ, Burke LM: Nutrition for power sports: middle-distance running, track cycling, rowing, canoeing/kayaking, and swimming. J Sports Sci 2011; 29(suppl 1):S79–S89.
17 Hawley JA, Burke LM: Carbohydrate availability and training adaptation: effects on cell metabolism. Exerc Sport Sci Rev 2010; 38:152–160.
18 Morton JP, Croft L, Bartlett JD, et al: Reduced carbohydrate availability does not modulate training-induced heat shock protein adaptations but does upregulate oxidative enzyme activity in human skeletal muscle. J Appl Physiol 2009;106:1513–1521.
19 Hawley JA, Burke LM, Phillips SM, Spriet LL: Nutritional modulation of training-induced skeletal muscle adaptations. J Appl Physiol 2011;110:834–845.
20 Guerra B, Guadalupe-Grau A, Fuentes T, et al: SIRT1, AMP-activated protein kinase phosphorylation and downstream kinases in response to a single bout of sprint exercise: influence of glucose ingestion. Eur J Appl Physiol 2010;109:731–743.
21 Cochran AJ, Little JP, Tarnopolsky MA, Gibala MJ: Carbohydrate feeding during recovery alters the skeletal muscle metabolic response to repeated sessions of high-intensity interval exercise in humans. J Appl Physiol 2010;108:628–636.
22 Coffey VG, Moore DR, Burd NA, et al: Nutrient provision increases signalling and protein synthesis in human skeletal muscle after repeated sprints. Eur J Appl Physiol 2011;111:1473–1483.
23 Edge J, Bishop D, Goodman C: Effects of chronic NaHCO3 ingestion during interval training on changes to muscle buffer capacity, metabolism, and short-term endurance performance. J Appl Physiol 2006;101:918–925.
24 Bishop DJ, Thomas C, Moore-Morris T, et al: Sodium bicarbonate ingestion prior to training improves mitochondrial adaptations in rats. Am J Physiol Endocrinol Metab 2010;299:E225–E233.
25 Derave W, Everaert I, Beeckman S, Baguet A: Muscle carnosine metabolism and beta-alanine supplementation in relation to exercise and training. Sports Med 2010;40:247–263.
26 Hill CA, Harris RC, Kim HJ, et al: Influence of beta-alanine supplementation on skeletal muscle carnosine concentrations and high intensity cycling capacity. Amino Acids 2007;32:225–233.
27 Hoffman J, Ratamess N, Kang J, et al: Effect of creatine and beta-alanine supplementation on performance and endocrine responses in strength/power athletes. Int J Sport Nutr Exerc Metab 2006;16:430–446.

Questions and Answers

Question 1: Dr. Gibala, HIT seems to result in a rapid and fast response of training adaptations. Could you explain the mechanism for that?

Answer: There are a number of different mechanisms. We know though that HIT stimulates many of the same molecular signalling pathways that are activated after endurance type training. So, from a molecular standpoint, much of the adaptive response appears quite similar. There are some differences and, for example, adaptations in fat metabolism appear to be a little bit slower. Given that HIT relies very heavily on carbohydrate for fuel, perhaps it is not surprising that the adaptations in carbohydrate metabolism are quite fast and the fat metabolism changes are a little more sluggish. That being said, within a few weeks of interval training, even of a very small volume, you can see increases in your capacity to oxidize fats in the muscle.

Question 2: Is HIT an exercise type for everybody?

Answer: Certainly any serious endurance athlete is already incorporating HIT into their normal training program. We have been looking at other populations including people with type 2 diabetes and metabolic syndrome. Even in these clinical populations, we see that they can perform interval training, and they can benefit. For example, 2 weeks of this type of training in type 2 diabetics lowered their 24-hour blood sugar levels, which we know is associated with positive health outcomes. In applying interval training to different groups, you need to properly monitor it and use some caution, but it can be widely applied to many different groups, and they can benefit.

Question 3: Are there any supplements that can further enhance the benefits of HIT?

Answer: In theory, any supplement that has been shown to acutely improve high-intensity performance could potentially augment adaptations to HIT, for example sodium bicarbonate, creatine or caffeine. Many of these supplements may be beneficial in theory, but the studies haven't been done to look at chronic training adaptations. There is a little bit of evidence that sodium bicarbonate ingestion chronically may improve performance even when subjects do work matched-work HIT protocols. So, even though the two groups of subjects did the exact same HIT protocol, chronic sodium bicarbonate ingestion resulted in a further improvement in performance. The mechanisms for that are not clear, but there is some evidence from rat studies that sodium bicarbonate actually improves the function of the mitochondria, and that might be a potential mechanism.

Question 4: You told me that you are doing HIT for yourself. Are you also taking supplements or food products?

Answer: No, I do not regularly consume supplements except for the caffeine in my morning coffee!

Dietary Strategies to Attenuate Muscle Loss during Recovery from Injury

Kevin D. Tipton

School of Sport, University of Stirling, Stirling, UK

Abstract

Injuries are an unavoidable aspect of participation in physical activity. Nutrition is important for optimal wound healing and recovery, but little information about nutritional support for injuries exists. Immediately following injury, wound healing begins with an inflammatory response. Excessive anti-inflammatory measures may impair recovery. Many injuries result in limb immobilization. Immobilization results in muscle loss due to increased periods of negative muscle protein balance from decreased basal muscle protein synthesis and resistance to anabolic stimuli, including protein ingestion. Oxidative capacity of muscle is also decreased. Nutrient and energy deficiencies should be avoided. Energy expenditure may be reduced during immobilization, but inflammation, wound healing and the energy cost of ambulation limit the reduction of energy expenditure. There is a theoretical rationale for leucine and omega-3 fatty acid supplementation to help reduce muscle atrophy. During rehabilitation and recovery from immobilization, increased activity, in particular resistance exercise will increase muscle protein synthesis and restore sensitivity to anabolic stimuli. Ample, but not excessive, protein and energy must be consumed to support muscle growth. During rehabilitation and recovery, nutritional needs are very much like those for any athlete desiring muscle growth. The most important consideration is to avoid malnutrition and to apply a risk/benefit approach.

Copyright © 2013 Nestec Ltd., Vevey/S. Karger AG, Basel

Introduction

Injuries are an unfortunate, but unavoidable part of sport. Injuries resulting from physical activity may lead to impairments in muscle size, strength and function, thus preventing optimal training and competitive success for an athlete. The negative aspects of injuries, particularly if it is prolonged or results in immobilization of a limb, are obvious. Injuries resulting from physical activity almost certainly will lead to decreased activity and loss of muscle mass, strength and function. Minimizing the impact of the injury and enhancing recovery from the injury are crucial for athletes, as well as other exercisers. Injuries resulting in reduced training and immobilization of the injured limb will lead to loss of muscle mass. Impairments in muscle function often follows muscle loss. One aspect of recovery that is often overlooked is nutrition. There has been much written about nutrition for injury, but surprisingly little is directly based on actual research. This review will focus primarily on acute, traumatic injuries and the problems associated with limb immobility and muscle loss, as well as nutritional countermeasures for these problems.

Nutritional Status

There is no question that poor nutritional status will impede healing and recovery from injury. In particular, protein and energy malnutrition exacerbates the inflammatory response and slows wound healing [1, 2]. The focus of this review primarily will be on healthy exercisers and athletes. Thus, malnourishment is unlikely to be an issue in most cases. In that context, this review will only refer to malnourishment in particular situations in which energy, protein and micronutrient intake may be poor prior to the injury.

Inflammation

Immediately following a severe injury, an inflammatory response is initiated. The inflammatory response is generally considered to be necessary for proper healing. This stage may last for a few hours up to several days depending on the injury [3]. As with many situations, too much of a good thing may be bad. Often, recommendations are made to decrease or even eliminate the inflammatory response. However, given that inflammation may be crucial for healing [3], elimination of the inflammation may not be ideal for healing. Unfortunately, not enough is known about the inflammatory process to be certain, but it seems sensible to avoid excessive inflammation. In that light, recommendations are made concerning fatty acid intake. In some very severe injuries, e.g. major burn injury, excessive inflammation may occur, particularly in patients that are otherwise metabolically compromised. However, most exercise-induced injuries, particularly in otherwise healthy exercisers and athletes, would not be severe enough for uncontrolled inflammation to be an issue [3]. Many recommend avoidance of too many omega-6 fatty acids and increased intake of omega-3 fatty acids. It should be noted that these recommendations seem to be based mostly on in vitro studies. Since omega-3 fatty acids are found primarily in fish oils, flax seed oils, walnuts, etc., supplements are often recommended. Omega-6 fatty acids are commonly found in vegetable oils, such as corn, sunflower, etc. Since we do not really understand the significance of the inflammatory process, nor do we know for certain that the omega-3 to omega-6 ratios in the diet actually impact inflammation following injury, no solid recommendations can be made. Thus, excessive supplementation of omega-3 fatty acids and decreased omega-6 fatty acids to decrease inflammation must be considered preliminary. Perhaps a 'first do no harm' or risk/benefit concept is the best recommendation. From that standpoint, decreasing sunflower, corn and cottonseed oil in the diet is not much of a burden and, if the theory is true, may help avoid excessive inflammation following an injury.

Loss of Muscle Mass during Immobility

Many exercise-induced injuries result in the necessity to immobilize a limb or otherwise reduce overall activity. If immobility is required following injury, the most obvious result is loss of muscle function resulting from changes in tendon function and loss of muscle mass [4–6]. Muscle protein balance, i.e. the balance between the rate of muscle protein synthesis and muscle protein breakdown, is the metabolic mechanism responsible for changes in muscle mass [7]. Negative net muscle protein balance results when the rate of muscle protein synthesis is exceeded by breakdown. Negative balance over any given time means that muscle protein is reduced resulting in muscle loss [7].

Negative net muscle protein balance with inactivity in humans leading to muscle loss is a decrease in the rate of muscle protein, particularly myofibrillar protein [5], synthesis [8]. Interestingly – perhaps unexpectedly to many [9] – protein breakdown also decreases, at least in humans [10]. The decrease in muscle protein synthesis is greater than the decrease in muscle protein breakdown, thus the muscle is in net negative protein balance. Clearly, nutritional interventions aimed at ameliorating muscle loss during injury-induced immobilization should focus on alleviating, as much as possible, the decrease in muscle protein synthesis such that negative periods of muscle protein balance are minimized. Given that ingestion of an amino acid source increases muscle protein synthesis resulting in positive net muscle protein balance [11], protein ingestion is the obvious nutritional intervention to help alleviate muscle loss. However, the impact of extra protein may be limited.

Anabolic Resistance

Another detrimental response to immobilization is that the response of muscle to anabolic stimuli is reduced. A recent investigation from Canada demonstrated that immobility decreases the ability of myofibrillar proteins to respond to increased availability of amino acids. Thus, despite the well-known ability for intake of a source of essential amino acids to increase muscle protein synthesis [11], the anabolic resistance will limit the anabolic impact of protein ingestion. However that study suggests that higher levels of blood amino acids, such as following greater protein intake, do have a greater impact on the rate of muscle protein synthesis than lower levels [5]. Thus, higher doses of protein intake may be important at any given meal, even if the overall protein intake is not necessarily increased. In healthy muscle, protein ingestion above ~20–25 g does not result in further stimulation of muscle protein synthesis [12]. The results presented above [5] could be interpreted to suggest that higher doses may be beneficial in immobilized muscle. However, this interpretation has not been investigated.

Another interesting concept in relation to protein intake during immobility is the type of protein that is synthesized in response to stimulation by protein ingestion. It is clear that myofibrillar protein is lost from immobilized muscle due to the aforementioned decrease in basal and amino acid-stimulated muscle protein synthesis [5]. Moreover, it is clear that protein ingestion stimulates both muscle myofibrillar and sarcoplasmic protein synthesis [13]. However, without exercise, at least resistance exercise, the stimulation of myofibrillar protein synthesis is transient and less than that of sarcoplasmic protein synthesis. Thus, it is not clear what the protein composition of muscle tissue would be as a result of protein ingestion during immobilization. Taken together, these studies could suggest that any stimulation of protein synthesis by extra protein ingestion may result in a greater proportion of sarcoplasmic, rather than myofibrillar, proteins. Thus, the overall beneficial effect of the protein ingestion may be less than often surmised.

Despite the inability of increased protein intake to alleviate muscle loss during immobility due to anabolic resistance, there is an intervention that could – at least potentially – decrease this resistance. Leucine is well known to increase protein synthesis in cell culture and rat studies [14–16]. Whereas leucine intake has been widely claimed to help increase muscle mass during resistance exercise training, the evidence is tenuous and unsubstantiated in human studies [17–19]. However, leucine may help overcome the resistance of muscle protein synthesis to anabolic stimuli. Leucine ingestion ameliorates muscle loss in rats during immobilization [20]. Moreover, studies in elderly humans show that the anabolic signaling pathways in muscle are inhibited, thus reducing protein synthesis [21]. However, the anabolic resistance may be overcome by increasing the leucine content of ingested protein [22]. To date, no study has specifically examined the impact of ingesting extra leucine with or without protein on muscle protein synthesis and muscle loss in immobilized human muscle. However, it is intriguing to consider and should be studied. Of course, the amount of leucine in relation to the protein and other details of such an intervention must be investigated in future studies.

There is new evidence, albeit rather limited, to suggest that fish oil supplementation may be important for muscle loss. A recent rat study demonstrated that fish oil supplementation may ameliorate muscle atrophy during immobilization [23]. Omega-3 fatty acids have long been recognized for their health effects, but only recently has evidence for increased muscle anabolism come to light. This effect seems to be mediated by attenuation of the immobilization-disturbed mTOR signaling pathways involved in translation initiation and muscle protein synthesis. Moreover, in humans, fish oil supplementation increases the response of muscle protein synthesis to the anabolic stimulation from amino acids [24]. Thus, the impact of fish oil supplementation during immobility for the limitation of muscle loss seems promising. However, as with many other potentially beneficial interventions, direct evidence in human studies is lacking.

Muscle Metabolism

Loss of muscle strength is not the only detrimental aspect of immobilization for athletes to consider. Recent evidence clearly demonstrates that muscle mitochondrial oxidative function and metabolic flexibility are impaired. Transcriptional downregulation of mitochondrial proteins, decreases in translational signaling pathways involved in mitochondrial biogenesis and declines in mitochondrial enzyme activities all result from immobilization [25]. Some of these changes occur as early as 48 h following initiation of inactivity. Nearly all aspects of mitochondrial function are impacted [25]. It is well known that inactivity leads to depressed insulin sensitivity [26]. The detrimental impact on glucose action may have much to do with the decreased GLUT4 content in immobilized muscle. Certainly, athletes and exercisers must consider these adverse changes to muscle oxidative and metabolic function during immobilization. Unfortunately, nutritional interventions that may alleviate these negative metabolic changes have not been investigated, thus recommendations are unclear. It is true that protein/amino acid ingestion concurrently with carbohydrate can in-

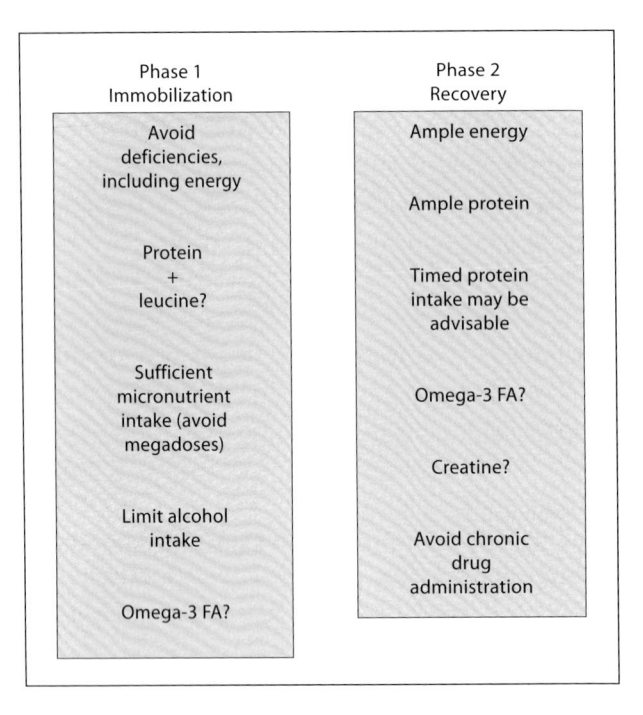

Phase 1 Immobilization	Phase 2 Recovery
Avoid deficiencies, including energy	Ample energy
	Ample protein
Protein + leucine?	Timed protein intake may be advisable
Sufficient micronutrient intake (avoid megadoses)	Omega-3 FA?
	Creatine?
Limit alcohol intake	Avoid chronic drug administration
Omega-3 FA?	

Fig. 1. Summary of nutritional suggestions for immobilization and rehabilitation phases after an activity-induced injury. FA = Fatty acids.

crease glucose disposal [27]. However, it is not clear how this approach would alleviate the decrease in insulin sensitivity of immobilized muscle. Clearly, it is crucial that athletes are as active as possible to avoid development of insulin resistance on a whole body level.

Energy Intake

Another important consideration during injury-induced immobilization is the appropriate energy intake (fig. 1). The first impulse of most injured athletes likely would be to reduce energy intake quite substantially. By necessity, the total energy expenditure likely will decrease during immobility. Depending on which limb is immobilized, a substantial decrease in total energy expenditure may develop voluntarily, because exercise is more difficult or less convenient, or by necessity as options are limited. However, there are factors to consider that should impact the magnitude of the necessary reduction. First, it is quite clear that during the healing process, energy expenditure is increased – particularly early on and if the injury is severe – by up to as much as 20%. So, whereas energy expenditure may still be less than during training, the total may not be as low as many would at first assume.

Another factor related to energy intake that may need to be considered by many injured athletes is the energy cost of getting around. If an injury results in the necessity to use crutches, the energy cost is dramatically increased. Ambulation with crutches results in energy expenditures in the range of 2–3× that of regular walking [28]. Thus, depending on how much crutching is done, energy intake may not need to go down by much at all.

The energy intake during immobilization also may have an impact on muscle protein synthesis. Care should be taken to ensure that any decrease in energy intake is not so much that optimal muscle protein synthesis is unsupported. It is clear that negative energy balance decreases muscle protein synthesis. Decreased synthesis is the major contributor to muscle loss. Clearly, the proper balance should be sought, but perhaps a wee bit of weight gain may be preferable to lack of energy to support proper muscle healing. That decision must be made after careful assessment and consultation between the nutritionist, athlete and coach.

Bone, Tendons and Ligaments

Muscle loss is the obvious focus during disuse stemming from injury. However, bone, tendons and ligaments are important for exercise performance and also are impacted negatively by immobilization. The connective tissue protein, collagen, is the primary component of tendons and ligaments. Decreased tendon collagen synthesis from immobilization results in changes in tendon mechanical properties. Collagen synthesis rates in tendon and muscle do not respond to increased amino acid levels [29], suggesting that protein feeding would have little impact on tendon healing. Bone collagen synthesis, an important aspect of bone healing, on the other hand, does respond to increased amino acid level. Certainly, sufficient intake of calcium and vitamin D is important for optimal healing. However, other aspects of tendon, bone and ligament healing in relation to collagen remain to be determined.

Conclusions and Recommendations

Limb immobilization from injuries has profound implications for muscle and tendon metabolism leading to loss of muscle size, strength and function. The negative impact on athletic performance and health is dramatic and must be reduced. Certainly, the most important nutritional consideration is to avoid deficiencies of any essential nutrient. During immobilization, ample energy and protein should be consumed. However, due to a resistance to the anabolic stimulus of the amino acids, the impact of excess protein intake is uncertain. However, it is unlikely to cause problems, so could perhaps be considered. Potentially, increased leucine intake may be helpful to diminish the anabolic resistance. An overly restrictive energy intake may actually be detrimental. Efforts to decrease the inflammatory response should be tempered unless it is clearly diagnosed as out of control or overly long. A cost/benefit approach may be best when considering supplementation of potentially beneficial countermeasures, such as leucine and omega-3 fatty acids. Moreover, there is a theoretical rationale for efficacy of other micronutrients, e.g. zinc and vitamin C, during healing, but little solid evidence. Whereas increasing food sources of these nutrients may be worthwhile, individual supplements are not likely the best recommendation. Finally, alcohol intake should be minimized, as should use of anti-inflammatories and antioxidant supplements.

Disclosure Statement

The author discloses no conflict of interest.

References

1 Demling RH: Nutrition, anabolism, and the wound healing process: an overview. Eplasty 2009;9:e9.
2 Arnold M, Barbul A: Nutrition and wound healing. Plast Reconstr Surg 2006;117:42S–58S.
3 Lin E, Kotani JG, Lowry SF: Nutritional modulation of immunity and the inflammatory response. Nutrition 1998;14:545–550.
4 Jones SW, Hill RJ, Krasney PA, et al: Disuse atrophy and exercise rehabilitation in humans profoundly affects the expression of genes associated with the regulation of skeletal muscle mass. FASEB J 2004;18:1025–1027.
5 Glover EI, Phillips SM, Oates BR, et al: Immobilization induces anabolic resistance in human myofibrillar protein synthesis with low and high dose amino acid infusion. J Physiol 2008;586:6049–6061.
6 de Boer MD, Maganaris CN, Seynnes OR, et al: Time course of muscular, neural and tendinous adaptations to 23 day unilateral lower-limb suspension in young men. J Physiol 2007;583:1079–1091.
7 Phillips SM, Glover EI, Rennie MJ: Alterations of protein turnover underlying disuse atrophy in human skeletal muscle. J Appl Physiol 2009;107:645–654.
8 Ferrando AA, Tipton KD, Bamman MM, Wolfe RR: Resistance exercise maintains skeletal muscle protein synthesis during bed rest. J Appl Physiol 1997;82:807–810.
9 Rennie MJ, Selby A, Atherton P, et al: Facts, noise and wishful thinking: muscle protein turnover in aging and human disuse atrophy. Scand J Med Sci Sports 2010;20:5–9.

10 Ferrando AA, Paddon-Jones D, Wolfe RR: Bed rest and myopathies. Curr Opin Clin Nutr Metab Care 2006;9:410–415.
11 Tipton KD, Ferrando AA, Phillips SM, et al: Postexercise net protein synthesis in human muscle from orally administered amino acids. Am J Physiol 1999;276:E628–E634.
12 Moore DR, Robinson MJ, Fry JL, et al: Ingested protein dose response of muscle and albumin protein synthesis after resistance exercise in young men. Am J Clin Nutr 2008;89:161–168.
13 Moore DR, Tang JE, Burd NA, et al: Differential stimulation of myofibrillar and sarcoplasmic protein synthesis with protein ingestion at rest and after resistance exercise. J Physiol 2009;587:897–904.
14 Anthony JC, Anthony TG, Layman DK: Leucine supplementation enhances skeletal muscle recovery in rats following exercise. J Nutr 1999;129:1102–1106.
15 Kimball SR, Jefferson LS: Regulation of global and specific mRNA translation by oral administration of branched-chain amino acids. Biochem Biophys Res Commun 2004;313:423–427.
16 Kimball SR, Jefferson LS: Role of amino acids in the translational control of protein synthesis in mammals. Semin Cell Dev Biol 2005;16:21–27.
17 Koopman R: Combined ingestion of protein and carbohydrate improves protein balance during ultra-endurance exercise. Am J Physiol Endocrinol Metab 2004;287:E712–E720.
18 Koopman R, Verdijk LB, Beelen M, et al: Co-ingestion of leucine with protein does not further augment post-exercise muscle protein synthesis rates in elderly men. Br J Nutr 2007;99:571–580.
19 Tipton KD, Elliott TA, Ferrando AA, et al: Stimulation of muscle anabolism by resistance exercise and ingestion of leucine plus protein. Appl Physiol Nutr Metab 2009;34:151–161.
20 Baptista IL, Leal ML, Artioli GG, et al: Leucine attenuates skeletal muscle wasting via inhibition of ubiquitin ligases. Muscle Nerve 2010;41:800–808.
21 Cuthbertson D, Smith K, Babraj J, et al: Anabolic signaling deficits underlie amino acid resistance of wasting, aging muscle. FASEB J 2005;19:422–424.
22 Katsanos CS, Kobayashi H, Sheffield-Moore M, et al: A high proportion of leucine is required for optimal stimulation of the rate of muscle protein synthesis by essential amino acids in the elderly. Am J Physiol Endocrinol Metab 2006;291:E381–E387.
23 You J-S, Park M-N, Song W, Lee Y-S: Dietary fish oil alleviates soleus atrophy during immobilization in association with Akt signaling to p70s6k and E3 ubiquitin ligases in rats. Appl Physiol Nutr Metab 2010;35:310–318.
24 Smith GI, Atherton P, Reeds DN, et al: Omega-3 polyunsaturated fatty acids augment the muscle protein anabolic response to hyperinsulinaemia-hyperaminoacidaemia in healthy young and middle-aged men and women. Clin Sci (Lond) 2011;121:267–278.
25 Abadi A, Glover EI, Isfort RJ, et al: Limb immobilization induces a coordinate down-regulation of mitochondrial and other metabolic pathways in men and women. PLoS One 2009;4:e6518.
26 Stuart CA, Shangraw RE, Prince MJ, et al: Bed-rest-induced insulin resistance occurs primarily in muscle. Metabolism 1988;37:802–806.
27 Manders RJ, Praet SF, Meex RC, et al: Protein hydrolysate/leucine co-ingestion reduces the prevalence of hyperglycemia in type 2 diabetic patients. Diabetes Care 2006;29:2721–2722.
28 Waters RL, Campbell J, Perry J: Energy cost of three-point crutch ambulation in fracture patients. J Orthop Trauma 1987;1:170–173.
29 Babraj JA, Cuthbertson DJ, Smith K, et al: Collagen synthesis in human musculoskeletal tissues and skin. Am J Physiol Endocrinol Metab 2005;289:E864–E869.

Questions and Answers

Question 1: Are there any nutritional strategies to prevent muscle mass loss without interfering with the healing process?

Answer: I think there probably are, mainly speculative evidence, but still worth trying. First of all, additional leucine with the diet might be important. There is some evidence that additional leucine may ameliorate the 'anabolic resistance' which occurs with immobilization of a limb. In other words, when an individual eats protein the muscle does not respond to the protein as it would in a healthy limb. So, there is some evidence that leucine can actually help ameliorate that or recover the feeding response. But I think there still needs to be further support to solidify that. Another thing I might try is to increase the omega-3 fatty acid content in the diet. There is some brand new evidence coming out that shows that omega-3 fatty acids enhance the muscle protein synthetic response to protein intake. That could be important in the situation where muscle protein synthesis is resistant to dietary protein intake. But these results need to be further tested in these specific situations before you can say for sure it is going to work.

Question 2: Is there a specific amount or a specific time that an individual should consume these omega-3 fatty acids?

Answer: The studies that were done supplemented 5 or 6 g per day, and of course that is assuming that the subjects already had a very low omega-3 fatty acid intake in the diet, which most people in North America and Europe do. And so, 5 or 6 g is something I would try if I were talking to an injured athlete and see if this might help. We do not know if this will really work, but there is not a whole lot of evidence suggesting that it will hurt anything. It is one of those risk/benefits things that you might want to try. Regarding the time of intake, because it is usually supplemented in the form of fish oil supplements, people tend to complain about a 'fishy' taste and maybe GI issues when you take it all at once. So, I would advise people to spread it throughout the day in smaller amounts.

Question 3: A lot of athletes assume when they are injured, they should lower their energy intake, is that correct?

Answer: That assumption is there among athletes, and to some extent it is probably valid. They certainly are not going to be training as hard, but their energy intake is going to be dependent on what they do for training. For instance, if they injure their leg and they are on crutches, they can still go to the gym and do work with the upper body and even the other leg. In fact, there is a good argument to do a lot of work with the other leg as there is evidence that there is a crossover effect to the uninjured limb. So, maybe if they are training hard, then that is one reason they should not decrease energy intake. Another reason is the injury in itself, depending on the severity of the injury, actually increases metabolism. The healing process costs energy, and so energy expenditure actually tends to go up immediately after the injury. Depending on the severity of the injury, basal metabolic rate can be increased by 50%, for example when there is a bone break. Maybe that keeps the energy expenditure slightly higher than most people think. Lastly, if the individual is on crutches, it actually takes 2–3 times more energy to get around than it does walking. So again, it is going to depend on the individual and how much they try to get around. For example, when I was injured, I was crutching into the office for 2 miles, so I spent a lot of energy doing that. The energy intake does not need to come down as much as some people may think. And the final factor is – muscle protein synthesis is an energetically expensive process. Thus, if you lower the energy intake too much, you can't have muscle protein synthesis increased as much as you should. Perhaps that is going to accelerate the loss of muscle when the limb is immobilized. I would argue that you are probably better off having an energy intake that is a little bit too much and maybe gain a little fat than losing even more muscle because you are restricting energy intake too much. People need to be careful about restricting energy intake.

Question 4: Why is leucine so important for muscle protein synthesis?

Answer: Leucine is a unique amino acid. Most amino acids are simply part of the polypeptide chain that makes a protein, but leucine seems to have a signaling aspect. Leucine actually turns on the metabolic and molecular pathways that result in greater muscle protein synthesis, so that is why leucine is critical in those situations. That may be the reason why leucine might work in those situations where the muscle is resistant to anabolic stimulation because it actually turns on those processes that are impaired by immobilization of the limb.

Question 5: Is whey protein more anabolic than casein due to the high leucine content?

Answer: We do not know that for sure. But I think there is mounting evidence that you can get a better muscle protein synthetic response after whey ingestion when compared with casein. Those studies are done mostly after exercise. So, we do not know whether this holds true after immobilization. But if you are going to take a supplement as part of that, maybe that is the best thing to do.

Question 6: What about casein, using it as a night protein?

Answer: I am not sure that has a whole lot of evidence. But I think you must take that into context of: 'Do I have room in my energy budget to have all this extra protein at night?' If you do, then maybe it is worth it. As far as an injured athlete is concerned, again, maybe you do not need to reduce the energy intake that much. I still would not pile on a lot of protein that gives a lot of energy, I would be careful about that.

The New Carbohydrate Intake Recommendations

Asker Jeukendrup

School of Sport and Exercise Sciences, University of Birmingham, Birmingham, UK

Abstract

Carbohydrate intake during prolonged exercise has been shown to increase endurance capacity and improve performance. Until recently, the advice was to ingest 30–60 g of carbohydrate per hour. The upper limit was based on studies that demonstrated that intakes greater than 60–70 g/h would not result in greater exogenous carbohydrate oxidation rates. The lower limit was an estimated guess of the minimum amount of carbohydrate required for ergogenic effects. In addition, the advice was independent of the type, the duration or the intensity of the activity as well as the level of athlete. Since 2004, significant advances in the understanding of the effects of carbohydrate intake during exercise have made it possible to be much more prescriptive and individual with the advice. Studies revealed that oxidation rates can reach much higher values (up to 105 g/h) when multiple transportable carbohydrates are ingested (i.e. glucose:fructose). It has also been observed that carbohydrate ingested during shorter higher intensity exercise (1 h, 80%VO$_{2max}$) can improve performance, although mechanisms are distinctly different. These findings resulted in new recommendations that are dependent on the duration and intensity of exercise and not only specify the quantity of carbohydrate to be ingested but also the type.

Copyright © 2013 Nestec Ltd., Vevey/S. Karger AG, Basel

Introduction

It has been known for some time that carbohydrate ingestion during exercise can increase exercise capacity and improve exercise performance [for reviews, see 1–4]. Although the exact mechanisms are still not completely understood, in general, two major mechanisms have been described and are either 'metabolic' or 'central' in origin.

The oldest and most established mechanisms relate to the effects of carbohydrate intake on metabolism. During exercise longer than 2 h, carbohydrate ingestion helps to maintain blood glucose concentrations and high rates of carbohydrate oxidation. This in turn, delays the onset of fatigue, extends time to exhaustion and can increase performance. The ergogenic effects of carbohydrate ingestion during exercise of high intensity (>75%VO$_{2max}$) and relatively short duration (~1 h) have a different origin and are not related to metabolism but reside in the central nervous system instead. Carbohydrate mouth rinses have been shown to result in performance improvements [5–9] suggesting that the beneficial effects of carbohydrate feeding during exercise are not confined to its conventional metabolic advantage but may also serve as a positive afferent signal capable of modifying motor output [10]. These effects are specific to carbohydrate and are independent of taste [11]. The receptors in the oral cavity have not yet been identified, and the exact role of various brain areas is not clearly understood. Further research is warranted to fully understand the separate taste transduction pathways for various carbohydrates and how these differ between mammalian species, particularly in humans. However, it has been convincingly demonstrated that carbohydrate is detected in oral cavity by yet unidentified receptors, and this can be linked to improvements in exercise performance [for review see 9]. New guidelines suggested here take these findings into account (fig. 1).

These results suggest that it is not necessary to ingest large amounts of carbohydrate during exercise lasting approximately 30 min to 1 h, and even a mouth rinse with a carbohydrate solution may be sufficient to get a performance benefit (fig. 1). In most conditions, the performance effects with the mouth rinse were similar to ingesting the drink, so there does not seem to be a disadvantage of taking the drink, although anecdotally athletes may complain of gastrointestinal distress when taking on board too much fluid. Of course, when the exercise is more prolonged (2 h or more), carbohydrate becomes a very important fuel, and it is essential to ingest carbohydrate. As will be discussed below, larger amounts of carbohydrate may be required for more prolonged exercise.

Different carbohydrates ingested during exercise may be utilized at different rates [2], but until a landmark publication in 2004 [12] it was believed that carbohydrate ingested during exercise could only be oxidized at a rate no higher than 1 g/min (60 g/h) independent of the type of carbohydrate. This is reflected in guidelines published by the American College of Sports Medicine which recommends that athletes should take between 30 and 60 g of carbohydrate during endurance exercise (>1 h) [13].

Duration	Carbohydrate intake advice		Type of carbohydrate	Nutritional training
30–75 min	Small amounts or mouth rinse	30 min	Single or multiple transportable carbohydrates	Nutritional training highly recommended
1–2 h	30 g/h	60 min	Single or multiple transportable carbohydrates	Nutritional training highly recommended
2–3 h	60 g/h	2 h	Single or multiple transportable carbohydrates	Nutritional training highly recommended
>2.5 h	90 g/h	>2.5 h	Multiple transportable carbohydrates	Nutritional training essential

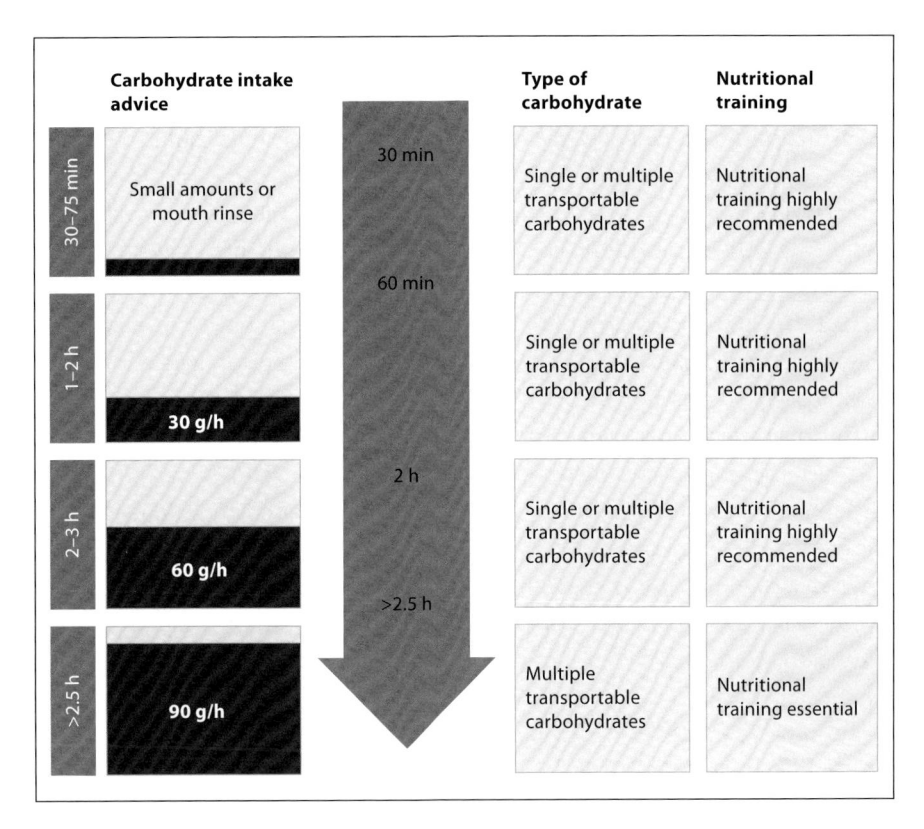

Fig. 1. Carbohydrate intake recommendations during exercise for exercise of different durations. These values are for high-level athletes and should be adjusted downwards for aspiring athletes.

Exogenous carbohydrate oxidation is most likely limited by the intestinal absorption of carbohydrates. It is believed that glucose uses a sodium-dependent transporter SGLT1 for absorption, which becomes saturated at a carbohydrate intake around 60 g/h. When glucose is ingested at this rate and another carbohydrate (fructose) that uses a different transporter is ingested simultaneously, oxidation rates that were well above 1 g/min (1.26 g/min) [12] can be observed. A series of studies followed in an attempt to work out the maximal rate of exogenous carbohydrate oxidation. In these studies, the rate of carbohydrate ingestion was varied and the types and combinations of carbohydrates differed. All studies confirmed that multiple transportable carbohydrates resulted in (up to 75%) higher oxidation rates than carbohydrates that use the SGLT1 transporter only [for reviews, see 1, 2]. Interestingly, such high oxidation rates could not only be achieved with carbohydrate ingested in a beverage but also as a gel [14] or a low-fat, low-protein, low-fiber energy bar [15].

Carbohydrate during Exercise and Performance: Dose Response

Very few well-controlled dose-response studies on carbohydrate ingestion during exercise and exercise performance have been published. Most of the older studies had serious methodological issues that made it difficult to establish a true dose response relationship between the amount of carbohydrate ingested and performance. Until recently, the conclusion seemed to be that you needed a minimum amount of carbohydrate (probably about 20 g/h based on one study), but it was assumed that there was no dose-response relationship [16].

In the last few years, evidence has been accumulating for a dose-response relationship between carbohydrate ingestion rates, exogenous carbohydrate oxidation rates and performance. In one recent carefully conducted study, endurance performance and fuel selection were measured during prolonged exercise while ingesting glucose (15, 30, and 60 g/h) [17]. Twelve subjects cycled for 2 h at 77%VO_{2peak} followed by a 20-km time trial. The results suggest a relationship between the dose of glucose ingested and improvements in endurance performance. The exogenous glucose oxidation increased with ingestion rate, and it is possible that an increase in exogenous carbohydrate oxidation is directly linked with, or responsible for, exercise performance [3, 4, 17, 18].

The superior effects of high intakes of multiple transportable carbohydrates seem to present themselves when the exercise duration is around 2.5 h or longer, and has not been demonstrated for shorter exercise bouts. Multiple transportable carbohydrates are essential to deliver these relatively large amounts of carbohydrate (>60 g/h). Multiple transportable carbohydrate ingestion does not result in increased exogenous carbohydrate oxidation or performance when ingested at rates below 60 g/h [19]. There are however no disadvantages to taking multiple transportable carbohydrates at rates below 60 g/h, and these carbohydrates are just as effective as a single source.

Training the Gut

Since the absorption of carbohydrate limits exogenous carbohydrate oxidation, and exogenous carbohydrate oxidation seems to be linked with exercise performance, an obvious potential strategy would be to increase the absorptive capacity of the gut. Anecdotal evidence in athletes would suggest that the gut is trainable and that individuals who regularly consume carbohydrate or have a high daily carbohydrate intake may also have an increased capacity to absorb it. Intestinal carbohydrate transporters can indeed be upregulated by exposing an animal to a high-carbohydrate diet [20]. To date, there is limited evidence in humans. A recent study by Cox et al. [21] investigated whether altering daily carbohydrate intake affects substrate oxidation and in particular exogenous carbohydrate oxidation. It was demonstrated that exogenous carbohydrate oxidation rates were higher after the high-carbohydrate diet (6.5 g/kg bodyweight per day; 1.5 g/kg bodyweight provided mainly as a carbohydrate supplement during training) for 28 days compared with a control diet (5 g/kg bodyweight per day). This study provided evidence that the gut is indeed adaptable, and this can be used as a practical method to increase exogenous carbohydrate oxidation. We recently suggested that this may be highly relevant to the endurance athlete, and may be a prerequisite for the first person to break the 2-hour marathon barrier [22].

Intermittent and Skill Sports

The vast majority of studies has been performed with endurance athletes performing continuous exercise. Most team sports have a highly intermittent nature with bursts of very high-intensity exercise followed by relatively low-intensity recovery periods. Besides this, performance in these sports is often dependent on other factors than maintenance of speed or power, and factors like agility, timing, motor skill, decision making, jumping, and sprinting may all play a role. Nevertheless, carbohydrate ingestion during exercise has also been shown to enhance endurance capacity in intermittent activities. A large number of studies have demonstrated that if carbohydrate is ingested during intermittent running, fatigue can be delayed and time to exhaustion can be increased [23–27].

More recently, studies have incorporated measurements of skill into their performance measurements. Currell et al. [28] developed a 90-min soccer simulation protocol that included measurements of skill, such as agility, dribbling, shooting and heading. The soccer players performed 90 min of intermittent exercise that mimicked their movement patterns during a game. During the 90 min, skill performance measurements were performed at regular intervals. Agility, dribbling and accuracy of shooting were all improved, but heading was not affected with carbohydrate ingestion. Other studies have found similar effects. Although typically a number of the skills measured in these studies were improved with carbohydrate feeding, the mechanisms behind these improvements are unknown and have not been studied in any detail.

It appears that carbohydrate intake during team sports and other sports with an element of skill has the potential to improve not only fatigue resistance but also the skill components of a sport, especially towards the end of a game. The practical challenge is often to find ways to ingest carbohydrate during a game within the rules of the sport.

Conclusions

There have been significant changes in the understanding of the role of carbohydrate during exercise in recent years, and this allows for more specific and more individualized advice with regard to carbohydrate ingestion during exercise. The new guidelines proposed take into account the duration (and intensity) of exercise, and advice is not restricted to the amount of carbohydrate, it also gives direction with respect to the type of carbohydrate. The recommendations presented here are derived mostly from studies with trained and well-trained athletes. Athletes who perform at absolute intensities that are lower will have lower carbohydrate oxidation rates and the amounts presented here should be adjusted accordingly. The recommended carbohydrate intake can be achieved by consuming drinks, gels, low-fat, low-protein and low-fiber solid foods (bars), and selection should be determined by personal preference. Athletes can adopt a mix and match strategy to achieve their carbohydrate intake goals. However, the carbohydrate intake should be balanced with a fluid intake plan, and it must be noted that solid foods and highly concentrated carbohydrate solutions have been shown to reduce fluid absorption. Although this can partly be prevented by using multiple transportable carbohydrates, this is something the athlete needs to consider when developing his/her nutrition strategy. Finally, it must be noted that most studies are based on findings in runners and cyclist, and more work is needed to establish the effects and underlying mechanisms of carbohydrate ingestion on skill components in intermittent team sports.

Disclosure Statement

The author received research funding from GlaxoSmithKline and Nestec for work that is relevant to this field. At the time of presenting and writing the author was employed by the University of Birmingham and he has since been employed by PepsiCo.

References

1 Jeukendrup A: Carbohydrate feeding during exercise. Eur J Sport Sci 2008;8:77–86.
2 Jeukendrup AE: Carbohydrate and exercise performance: the role of multiple transportable carbohydrates. Curr Opin Clin Nutr Metab Care 2010;13:452–457.
3 Jeukendrup AE, McLaughlin J: Carbohydrate ingestion during exercise: effects on performance, training adaptations and trainability of the gut. Nestle Nutr Inst Workshop Ser 2011;69:1–12, discussion 13–17.
4 Jeukendrup AE: Nutrition and endurance sports: running, cycling, triathlon. J Sports Sci, in press.
5 Carter JM, Jeukendrup AE, Jones DA: The effect of carbohydrate mouth rinse on 1-h cycle time trial performance. Med Sci Sports Exerc 2004;36:2107–2111.
6 Rollo I, Williams C, Gant N, Nute M: The influence of carbohydrate mouth rinse on self-selected speeds during a 30-min treadmill run. Int J Sport Nutr Exerc Metab 2008; 18:585–600.
7 Rollo I, Cole M, Miller R, Williams C: Influence of mouth rinsing a carbohydrate solution on 1-h running performance. Med Sci Sports Exerc 2010;42:798–804.
8 Fares EJ, Kayser B: Carbohydrate mouth rinse effects on exercise capacity in pre- and postprandial States. J Nutr Metab 2011;2011: 385962.
9 Jeukendrup AE, Chambers ES: Oral carbohydrate sensing and exercise performance. Curr Opin Clin Nutr Metab Care 2010;13: 447–451.
10 Gant N, Stinear CM, Byblow WD: Carbohydrate in the mouth immediately facilitates motor output. Brain Res 2010;1350:151–158.
11 Chambers ES, Bridge MW, Jones DA: Carbohydrate sensing in the human mouth: effects on exercise performance and brain activity. J Physiol 2009;587:1779–1794.
12 Jentjens RL, Moseley L, Waring RH, et al: Oxidation of combined ingestion of glucose and fructose during exercise. J Appl Physiol 2004;96:1277–1284.
13 Sawka MN, Burke LM, Eichner ER, et al: American College of Sports Medicine position stand. Exercise and fluid replacement. Med Sci Sports Exerc 2007;39:377–390.
14 Pfeiffer B, Stellingwerff T, Zaltas E, Jeukendrup AE: CHO oxidation from a CHO gel compared with a drink during exercise. Med Sci Sports Exerc 2010;42:2038–2045.
15 Pfeiffer B, Stellingwerff T, Zaltas E, Jeukendrup AE: Oxidation of solid versus liquid CHO sources during exercise. Med Sci Sports Exerc 2010;42:2030–2037.
16 Rodriguez NR, Di Marco NM, Langley S: American College of Sports Medicine position stand. Nutrition and athletic performance. Med Sci Sports Exerc 2009;41:709–731.
17 Smith JW, Zachwieja JJ, Peronnet F, et al: Fuel selection and cycling endurance performance with ingestion of [13C]glucose: evidence for a carbohydrate dose response. J Appl Physiol 2010;108:1520–1529.
18 Rowlands DS, Swift M, Ros M, Green JG: Composite versus single transportable carbohydrate solution enhances race and laboratory cycling performance. Appl Physiol Nutr Metab 2012;37:425–436.
19 Hulston CJ, Wallis GA, Jeukendrup AE: Exogenous CHO oxidation with glucose plus fructose intake during exercise. Med Sci Sports Exerc 2009;41:357–363.
20 Ferraris RP: Dietary and developmental regulation of intestinal sugar transport. Biochem J 2001;360:265–276.
21 Cox GR, Clark SA, Cox AJ, Halson SL, et al: Daily training with high carbohydrate availability increases exogenous carbohydrate oxidation during endurance cycling. J Appl Physiol 2010;109:126–134.
22 Stellingwerff T, Jeukendrup AE: Authors reply to Viewpoint by Joyner et al. entitled 'The Two-Hour Marathon: Who and When?' J Appl Physiol 2011;110:278–293.
23 Nicholas CW, Williams C, Lakomy HK, et al: Influence of ingesting a carbohydrate-electrolyte solution on endurance capacity during intermittent, high-intensity shuttle running. J Sports Sci 1995;13:283–290.
24 Nicholas CW, Nuttall FE, Williams C: The Loughborough Intermittent Shuttle Test: a field test that simulates the activity pattern of soccer. J Sports Sci 2000;18:97–104.

25 Foskett A, Williams C, Boobis L, Tsintzas K: Carbohydrate availability and muscle energy metabolism during intermittent running. Med Sci Sports Exerc 2008;40:96–103.
26 Davison GW, McClean C, Brown J, et al: The effects of ingesting a carbohydrate-electrolyte beverage 15 minutes prior to high-intensity exercise performance. Res Sports Med 2008;16:155–166.
27 Patterson SD, Gray SC: Carbohydrate-gel supplementation and endurance performance during intermittent high-intensity shuttle running. Int J Sport Nutr Exerc Metab 2007;17:445–455.
28 Currell K, Conway S, Jeukendrup AE: Carbohydrate ingestion improves performance of a new reliable test of soccer performance. Int J Sport Nutr Exerc Metab 2009;19:34–46.

Questions and Answers

Question 1: Carbohydrate provision maximizes performance. If you use carbohydrate blends (glucose, maltodextrin, fructose), you can actually absorb more carbohydrate during exercise. What are the practical limits for carbohydrate intake during exercise?

Answer: If you use a mix of different carbohydrates, we call them multiple transportable carbohydrates, you can achieve very high absorption and oxidation rates, and that has been shown to result in better performance during prolonged exercise (>2.5 h). It is important to realize that this only happens if you ingest relatively large amounts of carbohydrates. If you consume less than 60 g of carbohydrates per hour, you do not see these effects. You only see it if you push the carbohydrate intake higher than 60 g of carbohydrate per hour. We typically recommend around 90 g/h during this type of activity. That is actually quite a lot of carbohydrate to take on board during exercise, especially if you are not used to it. If you are unaccustomed, you can get some stomach discomfort, maybe some intestinal cramps. So the challenge is to ingest relatively large amounts of carbohydrate without causing gastrointestinal distress. The only way to get around this is to get used to it and use this practice in training. If you are planning to use this practice during a race, do not use this practice during the race for the very first time. Always practice the nutrition strategy in a training situation, and do it about once a week so the body is used to handling these large amounts of carbohydrate.

Question 2: Glucose availability in the mouth seems to directly improve performance capacity. Under what conditions would a little carbohydrate already have a practical relevance towards improve performance?

Answer: In some situations you do not need to actually ingest the carbohydrates to get the effect, but this is very specific to short-duration events. Most of the studies have investigated something around 60 min of all-out exercise, so maybe you see the effects from 30 up to 75 min. But it has to be an all-out effort for that period of time. Then, you can get these performance effects even with a simple mouth rinse. So, you can chose to rinse your mouth with a carbohydrate drink or you can chose to drink little bits of carbohydrate, and that should help your performance.

Question 3: Does this work only with glucose, or does this work with other sweeteners?

Answer: It does not work with any sweetener because in studies we and others used the sweetener as the placebo, and the carbohydrate improves performance compared with that placebo. So, it is a very specific effect of the carbohydrate and not of the sweetness. We have also done these studies with carbohydrates that have no taste and you can still see the performance effect. In fact, there are also studies that show that if you give a carbohydrate that is not sweet, it activates certain areas of the brain. So it is definitely a carbohydrate effect and not a sweetness effect.

Question 4: What is your personal and practical recommendation for carbohydrate intake during exercise for athletes?

Answer: The answer is: it depends. It depends on the level of athlete you are, and it depends on the type of event that you are involved in. Generally, if you are a higher level athlete who works out at higher absolute intensities, you probably need a little bit more carbohydrate. The event duration also matters. So if the event is very short you need smaller amounts of carbohydrate than when the event is very long. When the event is 2.5 h or longer and you really want optimal performance, you probably have to push the carbohydrate intake to as high as 90 g of carbohydrate per hour, use carbohydrates that contain multiple transportable carbohydrates. If you are in an event that is between, say 2–3 h, then you can probably get away with 60 g/h. If it is shorter, then you can go to 30 g/h. So, it really depends on what event you are looking at and what level of athlete you are.

Question 5: Is there also a difference if you consume carbohydrates during exercise as a solid food or as a liquid supplement?

Answer: That is a good question. We have recently done those studies where we compared drinks versus gels versus bars, and it turns out that it does not really matter how the carbohydrates are delivered. Gels with water are almost exactly the same as a sports drink. If you give carbohydrate bars with water, it is almost the same as a sport drink as well. But I think it is important that the bars or solid foods that you choose are low in fat, low in fiber and low in protein because as soon as you increase the content of those ingredients, you will slow down the delivery of the carbohydrate.

Role of Dietary Protein in Post-Exercise Muscle Reconditioning

Luc J.C. van Loon

Department of Human Movement Sciences, NUTRIM School for Nutrition, Toxicology and Metabolism, Maastricht University Medical Centre+, Maastricht, The Netherlands

Abstract

Dietary protein ingestion after exercise stimulates muscle protein synthesis, inhibits protein breakdown and, as such, stimulates net muscle protein accretion following resistance as well as endurance type exercise. Protein ingestion during and/or immediately after exercise has been suggested to facilitate the skeletal muscle adaptive response to each exercise session, resulting in more effective muscle reconditioning. A few basic guidelines can be defined with regard to the preferred type and amount of dietary protein and the timing by which protein should be ingested. Whey protein seems to be most effective to increase post-exercise muscle protein synthesis rates. This is likely attributed to its rapid digestion and absorption kinetics and specific amino acid composition. Ingestion of approximately 20 g protein during and/or immediately after exercise is sufficient to maximize post-exercise muscle protein synthesis rates. Additional ingestion of large amounts of carbohydrate does not further increase post-exercise muscle protein synthesis rates when ample protein is already ingested. Dietary protein should be ingested during and/or immediately after cessation of exercise to allow muscle protein synthesis rates to reach maximal levels. Future research should focus on the impact of the timing of protein provision throughout the day on the adaptive response to more prolonged exercise training.

Copyright © 2013 Nestec Ltd., Vevey/S. Karger AG, Basel

Skeletal Muscle Plasticity

It has been well established that nutrition is a key factor in determining exercise performance capacity. Many recreational and professional athletes apply short-term nutritional interventions to maximize performance capacity. Specifically designed sports nutrition products have been developed and are widely used among athletes in an effort to compensate for the metabolic demands imposed upon by competition. However, as many athletes will reach their limits with regard to training volume and intensity, proper dietary practice to support the adaptive response to more prolonged training has become of key importance. A greater adaptive response to the many training hours spent in the gym or on the field would improve training efficiency and, as such, improve performance capacity. The latter has renewed the interest among athletes, coaches, and scientists in the role of the diet and nutritional modulation in optimizing training efficiency. This chapter will provide an overview on the impact of dietary protein administration following exercise on the skeletal muscle adaptive response.

Skeletal muscle tissue easily adapts to structural changes in muscle (dis)use. This level of adaptability, often referred to as muscle tissue plasticity, becomes most evident when we compare the phenotypic response to more prolonged resistance versus endurance type exercise training. Simply compare the physique of a professional weightlifter with that of a marathon runner. The capacity of skeletal muscle tissue to adapt to changes in its use (or disuse) is a consequence of the fact that skeletal muscle tissue turns over at a rate of ~1–2% per day. Throughout a normal day, muscle protein synthesis rates may vary considerably and range between 0.04 and 0.14% per hour. The latter largely depends on food intake and habitual physical activity, the two main anabolic stimuli. Food intake, or rather protein ingestion, directly elevates muscle protein synthesis rates. Following protein digestion and absorption, the rise in plasma essential amino acid (EAA) concentrations (with leucine in particular) stimulates muscle protein synthesis rates. Such a postprandial increase in muscle protein synthesis rate will typically last for 2–3 h after meal ingestion. It is obvious that amino acids are much more than simply precursors of de novo muscle protein synthesis, as they also act as strong nutritional signaling molecules regulating multiple cellular processes.

In addition to food intake, physical activity represents another potent anabolic stimulus. A single bout of physical activity or exercise will strongly increase muscle protein synthesis rates, an effect that can persist for more than 24 h. The stimulating properties of food intake and physical activity on muscle protein synthesis throughout the day compensate for daily protein breakdown, thereby allowing skeletal muscle maintenance throughout most of our lifespan.

Dietary Protein Ingestion following Exercise

For any athlete in training, the main goal is to adapt to the exercise training regimen, thereby allowing structural changes to occur that will allow him or her to obtain a higher performance level. For muscle tissue reconditioning to occur, muscle protein synthesis and breakdown rates need to be increased over a given period of time. A single session of exercise will increase skeletal muscle protein synthesis and, to a lesser extent, muscle protein breakdown rates, thereby improving muscle protein balance [1]. Of course, differences will exist in the specific sets of muscle proteins that are expressed following various types of exercise. Whereas resistance type exercise mainly stimulates the expression of myofibrillar proteins, endurance type exercise mainly increases the expression of proteins involved in oxidative metabolism, thereby allowing sport-specific muscle adaptation [2]. Though exercise will improve muscle protein balance, net balance will remain negative in the absence of food intake. Consequently, nutrition is required for proper muscle reconditioning and to allow muscle hypertrophy to occur. It is here that the synergy between exercise and nutrition becomes evident. When protein is ingested following a single bout of exercise, muscle protein synthesis rates are increased to a much higher level. Furthermore, muscle protein synthesis rates also remain elevated for an extended period of time when compared with a normal postprandial response [3]. More recent work from our laboratory shows that exercise performed prior to food intake will allow more of the ingested protein to be used for de novo muscle protein synthesis [4]. The latter clearly shows that the metabolic fate of ingested protein largely depends on the activity performed prior to food consumption. These stimulating effects of exercise on the postprandial muscle protein synthetic response seem to be long-lived, with the protein synthetic response to protein ingestion still being elevated 24 h after the last exercise session [5]. There is a big challenge ahead to investigate how we can use this information to define dietary regimens that will optimize post-exercise muscle protein reconditioning. So far, there are surprisingly little data on the impact of the various nutritional factors that can modulate the post-exercise muscle protein synthetic response. However, some data have been acquired on the amount and type of dietary protein and the desired timing of protein ingestion that will optimize post-exercise muscle protein synthesis rates.

Amount of Dietary Protein

Protein/amino acid administration is required to stimulate post-exercise muscle protein synthesis rates, suppress the exercise-induced increase in protein breakdown and, as such, to achieve a positive muscle protein balance [6]. Tipton et al. [7] showed that ingestion of either mixed amino acids (MAA) or EAA only effectively stimulated post-exercise muscle protein synthesis rates. Since then,

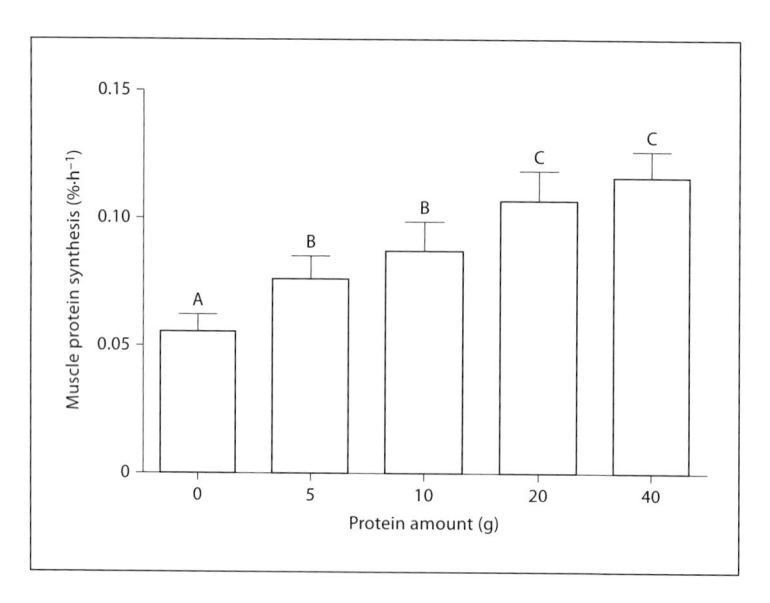

Fig. 1. Dose-reponse relationship between the amount of protein ingested and post-exercise muscle protein synthesis rates. Values represent means ± SEM. Means with different letters are significantly different from each other. Figure redrawn from Moore et al. [18].

numerous other studies have shown that amino acid and/or protein administration increases muscle protein synthesis rates following resistance type exercise [7–14] as well as endurance type exercise activities [15–17]. In short, post-exercise protein ingestion is required to facilitate subsequent muscle reconditioning.

Previously, Tipton et al. [7] showed that ingestion of 40 g MAA or EAA effectively stimulated post-exercise muscle protein synthesis. Since the ingestion of 40 g MAA or 40 g EAA resulted in a similar net protein balance, it was suggested that it might not be necessary to ingest nonessential amino acids during immediate post-exercise recovery. Follow-up studies assessed the impact of ingesting merely 6 g EAA (which would translate to ~12 g protein) with and without carbohydrate, and showed that this amount was also effective in stimulating post-exercise muscle protein synthesis. However, ingestion of such a small amount of EAA after exercise resulted in a positive net protein balance for up to 2 h only, after which net protein balance became negative again [9]. The latter implies that ingestion of such a small amount of amino acids is insufficient to remain in an anabolic state. Recently, Moore et al. [18] conducted a dose-response study to investigate the relationship between the amount of dietary protein ingested and subsequent post-exercise muscle protein synthesis rates (fig. 1). The fractional mixed muscle protein synthetic rate increased with the ingestion of greater amounts of protein, reaching maximal synthesis rates following ingestion of 20 g intact (egg) protein, which provides approximately 8.6 g EAA. The authors speculated that athletes should ingest such an amount of dietary protein 5–6 times daily to allow maximal stimulation of skeletal muscle protein synthesis rate throughout the day. More work is needed to assess the dose-response relationship between the amount of protein and the expression of different sets of protein during recovery from various types of exercise.

Source of Dietary Protein

Various dietary protein sources have been used in studies investigating the impact of post-exercise protein provision on the muscle protein synthetic response. Improvements in post-exercise protein balance and/or greater muscle protein synthesis rates have been reported following the ingestion of whey protein [8], casein protein [8], soy protein [19], casein protein hydrolysate [11, 20], egg protein [18], and whole-milk and/or fat-free milk [19, 21]. So what protein source maximizes post-exercise muscle protein synthesis rates? That question is difficult to answer as it is impossible to compare protein synthesis rates between these studies. Differences in the type, intensity, and duration of the exercise performed prior to protein ingestion, the duration of the recovery period that is being assessed, and the amount, type, and timing of the protein administered, modulate the post-exercise muscle protein synthetic rate. Only a few studies have compared differences in the post-exercise muscle protein synthetic response following the ingestion of protein sources.

Milk-derived proteins, such as whey and casein, seem to offer an anabolic advantage over soy protein [19, 22]. Casein and whey protein have distinct anabolic properties, which can be attributed to differences in digestion and absorption kinetics as well as amino acid composition [23, 24]. Whey protein is a soluble protein that is rapidly digested and absorbed following ingestion. In contrast, intact casein tends to clot in the stomach after ingestion, thereby delaying digestion and absorption, resulting in a slower release of protein-derived amino acids in the circulation [25]. The faster, more transient rise in plasma amino acid concentrations following whey ingestion generally leads to a more pronounced stimulation of muscle protein synthesis rate during the first few hours following ingestion when compared with casein ingestion [23]. The latter is likely also attributed to the higher leucine content of whey versus casein protein [22, 24]. However, these findings do not imply that additional leucine supplementation can further augment the post-exercise muscle protein synthetic response to food intake. Previously, we have reported that coingestion of crystalline leucine does not further increase post-exercise muscle protein synthesis rates when ample protein is already ingested [11, 20, 26].

More work is required to assess the impact of digestion and absorption kinetics and amino acid composition of a protein source on stimulating muscle protein reconditioning following resistance or endurance type exercise activities.

Carbohydrate Ingestion

Carbohydrate ingestion following exercise inhibits exercise-stimulated muscle protein breakdown, but does not affect muscle protein synthesis rates [8]. Though carbohydrate ingestion can improve muscle protein balance, net balance will remain negative without protein intake. The inhibitory effect of carbohydrate ingestion on protein breakdown has been attributed to the concomitant rise in circulating insulin. Consequently, many athletes involved in resistance type exercise training often ingest large quantities of carbohydrate with protein following cessation of exercise. Though the combined ingestion of protein with large amounts of carbohydrate is generally advocated in popular media, there is little scientific support to suggest that coingestion of carbohydrate will augment net muscle protein accretion following exercise. In an attempt to assess whether carbohydrate coingestion is required to maximize post-exercise muscle protein synthesis, we observed no benefit of the coingestion of either a small or large amount of carbohydrate on post-exercise muscle protein synthesis rates under conditions where ample protein is ingested [10]. Though carbohydrate coingestion does not seem to be required to maximize post-exercise muscle protein synthesis rates, it is likely that some carbohydrate can attenuate the post-exercise rise in muscle protein breakdown rate, thereby improving net protein balance [8]. Furthermore, as muscle glycogen content can be reduced by 30–40% following a single session of resistance type exercise [27], some carbohydrate coingestion may be preferred when these athletes wish to allow full muscle glycogen repletion to maintain exercise performance capacity.

Timing of Dietary Protein Ingestion

Besides the amount and type of protein, the timing of protein ingestion forms another key factor modulating post-exercise muscle anabolism. Levenhagen et al. [28] reported a more positive post-exercise net protein balance after consuming a (protein containing) supplement immediately after cessation of exercise as opposed to 3 h later. Furthermore, recent studies suggest that protein coingestion prior to and/or during exercise may further stimulate post-exercise muscle protein accretion [14, 29]. Tipton et al. [14] were the first to show that amino acid in-

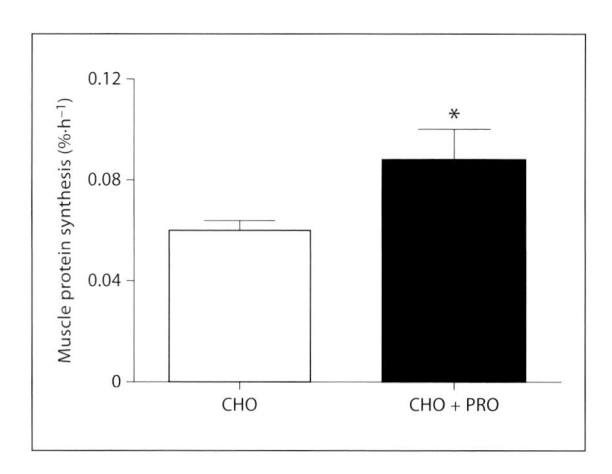

Fig. 2. Dietary protein ingestion prior to and during resistance type exercise stimulates muscle protein synthesis during exercise. Fractional synthesis rate of mixed muscle protein during exercise following carbohydrate (CHO) or carbohydrate plus protein (CHO+PRO) ingestion. Values represent means ± SEM. Asterisk denotes significant difference vs. CHO. Figure redrawn from Beelen et al. [29].

gestion prior to, as opposed to after, exercise augments net muscle protein accretion during subsequent post-exercise recovery. The stimulating effects of protein or amino acid supplementation prior to exercise on muscle protein synthesis after exercise have previously been attributed to a more rapid supply of amino acids during the acute stages of post-exercise recovery. In addition, we speculated that protein ingestion prior to and/or during resistance type exercise could already stimulate muscle protein synthesis during exercise conditions, allowing muscle protein synthesis rates to be elevated for an extended duration. In a recent study, we confirmed that coingestion of protein with carbohydrate before and during 2 h of intermittent resistance type exercise stimulates muscle protein synthesis during exercise [29] (fig. 2). The impact of protein coingestion on mixed muscle protein synthesis during exercise may be restricted to intermittent, resistance-type exercise activities [29]. It remains to be determined if protein ingestion before and/or during exercise can also increase muscle protein synthesis rates during continuous endurance type exercise. Preliminary findings suggest that protein coingestion stimulates muscle protein synthesis also during more prolonged endurance type exercise [30]. More work is needed to address the relevance of the potential to stimulate muscle protein synthesis during exercise, thereby creating a larger time frame for muscle protein synthesis rates to be increased.

For obvious methodological issues, post-exercise muscle reconditioning has hardly been studied during overnight sleep. Recently, we evaluated the impact of exercise performed in the evening on muscle protein synthesis during subsequent

Table 1. Practical recommendations for the athlete regarding dietary protein consumption during and/or immediately after an exercise session

– Provide sufficient protein (20–25 g) with each main meal
– Ingest 20–25 g dietary protein during or immediately after an exercise session
– Whey forms an excellent source of dietary protein to promote post-exercise recovery
– Coingest carbohydrate based on the need to replete liver and muscle glycogen stores
– Coingest some protein during more prolonged exercise (~0.10 g/kg bodyweight per hour)

overnight recovery [31]. Though an increase in muscle protein synthesis rates was observed during the first few hours of post-exercise recovery, muscle protein synthesis rates remained unexpectedly low during subsequent overnight sleep. Clearly, though post-exercise protein ingestion stimulates muscle protein synthesis during the acute stages of post-exercise recovery, these elevated muscle protein synthesis rates are not maintained during subsequent overnight recovery. It will be of interest to explore the impact of protein ingestion prior to or even during sleep on subsequent overnight muscle protein synthesis rates [32]. Overall, more work is needed to address the impact of the distribution of dietary protein throughout the day on prolonged training responses.

Conclusion

Protein ingestion following resistance or endurance type exercise will facilitate the skeletal muscle adaptive response to each successive exercise bout, resulting in more effective muscle reconditioning. Whey protein seems to be the most effective in stimulating acute post-exercise muscle protein synthesis. Ingestion of ~20 g protein during and/or immediately after each exercise bout is sufficient to allow maximal post-exercise muscle protein synthesis rates (table 1). Co-ingestion of large amounts of carbohydrate is not required to maximize post-exercise muscle protein accretion when ample protein is already ingested. A healthy diet with smart timing of the dietary protein ingestion after each bout of exercise will likely improve the skeletal muscle adaptive response to more prolonged exercise training.

Disclosure Statement

The author declares that no financial or other conflict of interest exists in relation to the content of the chapter.

References

1 Phillips SM, Tipton KD, Aarsland A, et al: Mixed muscle protein synthesis and breakdown after resistance exercise in humans. Am J Physiol 1997;273:E99–E107.
2 Wilkinson SB, Phillips SM, Atherton PJ, et al: Differential effects of resistance and endurance exercise in the fed state on signalling molecule phosphorylation and protein synthesis in human muscle. J Physiol 2008;586: 3701–3717.
3 Moore DR, Tang JE, Burd NA, et al: Differential stimulation of myofibrillar and sarcoplasmic protein synthesis with protein ingestion at rest and after resistance exercise. J Physiol 2009;587:897–904.
4 Pennings B, Koopman R, Beelen M, et al: Exercising before protein intake allows for greater use of dietary protein-derived amino acids for de novo muscle protein synthesis in both young and elderly men. Am J Clin Nutr 2010;93:322–331.
5 Burd NA, West DW, Moore DR, et al: Enhanced amino acid sensitivity of myofibrillar protein synthesis persists for up to 24 h after resistance exercise in young men. J Nutr 2011;141:568–573.
6 Biolo G, Tipton KD, Klein S, Wolfe RR: An abundant supply of amino acids enhances the metabolic effect of exercise on muscle protein. Am J Physiol 1997;273:E122–E129.
7 Tipton KD, Ferrando AA, Phillips SM, et al: Postexercise net protein synthesis in human muscle from orally administered amino acids. Am J Physiol 1999;276:E628–E634.
8 Borsheim E, Cree MG, Tipton KD, et al: Effect of carbohydrate intake on net muscle protein synthesis during recovery from resistance exercise. J Appl Physiol 2004;96:674–678.
9 Borsheim E, Tipton KD, Wolf SE, Wolfe RR: Essential amino acids and muscle protein recovery from resistance exercise. Am J Physiol Endocrinol Metab 2002;283:E648–E657.
10 Koopman R, Beelen M, Stellingwerff T, et al: Coingestion of carbohydrate with protein does not further augment postexercise muscle protein synthesis. Am J Physiol Endocrinol Metab 2007;293:E833–E842.
11 Koopman R, Wagenmakers AJ, Manders RJ, et al: Combined ingestion of protein and free leucine with carbohydrate increases postexercise muscle protein synthesis in vivo in male subjects. Am J Physiol Endocrinol Metab 2005;288:E645–E653.
12 Miller SL, Tipton KD, Chinkes DL, et al: Independent and combined effects of amino acids and glucose after resistance exercise. Med Sci Sports Exerc 2003;35:449–455.
13 Rasmussen BB, Tipton KD, Miller SL, et al: An oral essential amino acid-carbohydrate supplement enhances muscle protein anabolism after resistance exercise. J Appl Physiol 2000;88:386–392.
14 Tipton KD, Rasmussen BB, Miller SL, et al: Timing of amino acid-carbohydrate ingestion alters anabolic response of muscle to resistance exercise. Am J Physiol Endocrinol Metab 2001;281:E197–E206.
15 Gibala MJ: Protein metabolism and endurance exercise. Sports Med 2007;37:337–340.
16 Howarth KR, Moreau NA, Phillips SM, Gibala MJ: Coingestion of protein with carbohydrate during recovery from endurance exercise stimulates skeletal muscle protein synthesis in humans. J Appl Physiol 2009; 106:1394–1402.
17 Levenhagen DK, Carr C, Carlson MG, et al: Postexercise protein intake enhances whole-body and leg protein accretion in humans. Med Sci Sports Exerc 2002;34:828–837.
18 Moore DR, Robinson MJ, Fry JL, et al: Ingested protein dose response of muscle and albumin protein synthesis after resistance exercise in young men. Am J Clin Nutr 2009;89:161–168.
19 Wilkinson SB, Tarnopolsky MA, Macdonald MJ, et al: Consumption of fluid skim milk promotes greater muscle protein accretion after resistance exercise than does consumption of an isonitrogenous and isoenergetic soy-protein beverage. Am J Clin Nutr 2007; 85:1031–1040.
20 Koopman R, Verdijk L, Manders RJ, et al: Co-ingestion of protein and leucine stimulates muscle protein synthesis rates to the same extent in young and elderly lean men. Am J Clin Nutr 2006;84:623–632.
21 Elliot TA, Cree MG, Sanford AP, et al: Milk ingestion stimulates net muscle protein synthesis following resistance exercise. Med Sci Sports Exerc 2006;38:667–674.

22 Tang JE, Moore DR, Kujbida GW, et al: Ingestion of whey hydrolysate, casein, or soy protein isolate: effects on mixed muscle protein synthesis at rest and following resistance exercise in young men. J Appl Physiol 2009;107:987–992.
23 Boirie Y, Dangin M, Gachon P, et al: Slow and fast dietary proteins differently modulate postprandial protein accretion. Proc Natl Acad Sci USA 1997;94:14930–14935.
24 Pennings B, Boirie Y, Senden JM, et al: Whey protein stimulates postprandial muscle protein accretion more effectively than do casein and casein hydrolysate in older men. Am J Clin Nutr 2011;93:997–1005.
25 Koopman R, Crombach N, Gijsen AP, et al: Ingestion of a protein hydrolysate is accompanied by an accelerated in vivo digestion and absorption rate when compared with its intact protein. Am J Clin Nutr 2009;90:106–115.
26 Koopman R, Verdijk LB, Beelen M, et al: Co-ingestion of leucine with protein does not further augment post-exercise muscle protein synthesis rates in elderly men. Br J Nutr 2008;99:571–580.
27 Koopman R, Manders RJ, Jonkers RA, et al: Intramyocellular lipid and glycogen content are reduced following resistance exercise in untrained healthy males. Eur J Appl Physiol 2006;96:525–534.
28 Levenhagen DK, Gresham JD, Carlson MG, et al: Postexercise nutrient intake timing in humans is critical to recovery of leg glucose and protein homeostasis. Am J Physiol Endocrinol Metab 2001;280:E982–E993.
29 Beelen M, Koopman R, Gijsen AP, et al: Protein coingestion stimulates muscle protein synthesis during resistance-type exercise. Am J Physiol Endocrinol Metab 2008;295:E70–E77.
30 Beelen M, Zorenc A, Pennings B, et al: Impact of protein coingestion on muscle protein synthesis during continuous endurance type exercise. Am J Physiol Endocrinol Metab 2011;300:E945–E954.
31 Beelen M, Tieland M, Gijsen AP, et al: Coingestion of carbohydrate and protein hydrolysate stimulates muscle protein synthesis during exercise in young men, with no further increase during subsequent overnight recovery. J Nutr 2008;138:2198–2204.
32 Groen BB, Res PT, Pennings B, et al: Intragastric protein administration stimulates overnight muscle protein synthesis in elderly men. Am J Physiol Endocrinol Metab 2011;302:E52–E60.

Questions and Answers

Question 1: Are there large differences in the post-exercise muscle protein synthesis response regarding different types of proteins?

Answer: Yes. If you perform exercise, your protein synthesis will increase, and the types of protein that you are using will have an effect on the post-exercise muscle protein synthesis rates. For example, if you use animal-based proteins, generally the response seems to be greater than when you use plant-derived proteins.

Question 2: So where's the big difference between whey protein and casein?

Answer: If you go for milk protein, which is composed of both whey as well as casein, you will see that whey protein ingestion following exercise actually leads to a greater post-exercise muscle protein synthetic response when compared with casein protein.

Question 3: What protein source do you recommend to athletes?

Answer: For post-exercise recovery, you should actually have a protein that is rapidly digested and absorbed, and subsequently also has a high leucine content. So, whey protein would be one of the best proteins for post-exercise recovery.

Question 4: Is there a specific amount of protein that should be ingested following exercise?

Answer: There are a lot of studies still lacking, and it likely depends on the athlete and the type of exercise, but basically 20 g of protein should be enough to maximize post-exercise muscle protein synthesis rates. We don't necessarily need to ingest more than 20 g, and that's about the amount of protein you will find in a normal meal.

Question 5: Should endurance athletes worry about protein ingestion?

Answer: Every athlete should worry about protein ingestion. For example, endurance athletes also see an increase in protein synthesis following exercise, and to allow muscle reconditioning they also have to ingest dietary protein.

Question 6: Should they take supplements or just normal food?

Answer: Not necessarily supplements, but supplements sometimes are very practical because you can ingest them immediately after an exercise bout, but if you time your meals well, you can also have your meal (containing protein) after an exercise session.

Question 7: Do you take any supplements?

Answer: Yes, sometimes when I can't time my meals well, I take protein supplements following an exercise session.

Nutritional Support to Maintain Proper Immune Status during Intense Training

Michael Gleeson

School of Sport, Exercise and Health Sciences, Loughborough University, Loughborough, UK

Abstract

Prolonged exercise and heavy training are associated with depressed immune function which can increase the risk of picking up minor infections. To maintain robust immunity, athletes should eat a well-balanced diet sufficient to meet their energy, carbohydrate, protein, and micronutrient requirements. Dietary deficiencies of protein and specific micronutrients have long been associated with immune dysfunction and an adequate intake of iron, zinc, and vitamins A, D, E, B_6 and B_{12} is particularly important in the maintenance of immune function. Consuming carbohydrate during prolonged strenuous exercise attenuates rises in stress hormones and appears to limit the degree of exercise-induced immune depression. Similar effects can be seen with daily ingestion of high-dose antioxidant vitamin supplements, though concerns have been expressed that excessive antioxidant intake may impair exercise training adaptations. It is safe to say with reasonable confidence that individual amino acids, colostrum, Echinacea, and zinc are unlikely to boost immunity or reduce infection risk in athletes. The ingestion of carbohydrate during exercise and daily consumption of probiotic and plant polyphenol (e.g. quercetin)-containing supplements or foodstuffs (e.g. non-alcoholic beer) currently offer the best chance of success. This approach is likely to be most effective for individuals who are particularly prone to illness. Copyright © 2013 Nestec Ltd., Vevey/S. Karger AG, Basel

Introduction

Athletes who engage in intense training or who have recently competed in endurance race events appear to be at increased risk of developing symptoms of minor respiratory illness [1]. The most common illnesses in athletes are viral infections of the upper respiratory tract (i.e. the common cold), but athletes can also develop similar symptoms (e.g. sore throat) due to allergy or

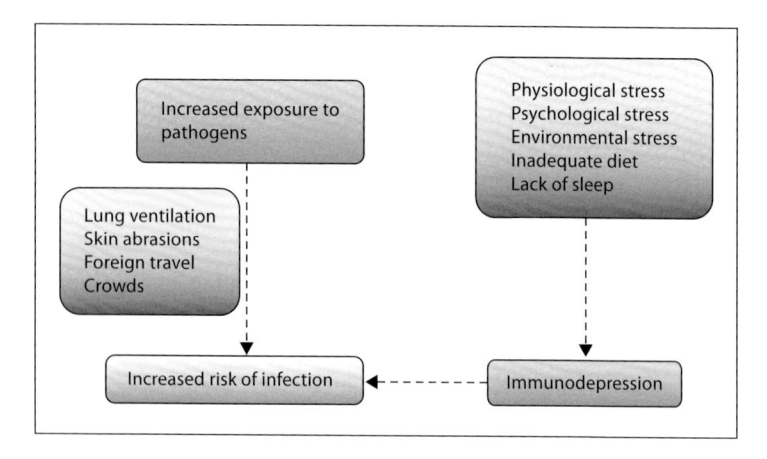

```
┌─────────────────────────────────────────────────────────────┐
│                                    ┌──────────────────────┐ │
│         ┌──────────────────────┐   │ Physiological stress │ │
│         │ Increased exposure to│   │ Psychological stress │ │
│         │     pathogens        │   │ Environmental stress │ │
│         └──────────────────────┘   │ Inadequate diet      │ │
│  ┌──────────────────┐              │ Lack of sleep        │ │
│  │ Lung ventilation │              └──────────────────────┘ │
│  │ Skin abrasions   │                                       │
│  │ Foreign travel   │                                       │
│  │ Crowds           │                                       │
│  └──────────────────┘                                       │
│         ┌──────────────────────┐   ┌──────────────────────┐ │
│         │Increased risk of infection│◄──│ Immunodepression │ │
│         └──────────────────────┘   └──────────────────────┘ │
└─────────────────────────────────────────────────────────────┘
```

Fig. 1. Causes of increased infection risk in athletes.

inflammation caused by inhalation of cold, dry or polluted air [2]. In themselves, these symptoms are generally trivial, but no matter whether the cause is infectious or allergic inflammation, they can cause an athlete to interrupt training, underperform or even miss an important competition. Prolonged bouts of strenuous exercise have been shown to result in transient depression of white blood cell functions, and it is suggested that such changes create an 'open window' of decreased host protection, during which viruses and bacteria can gain a foothold, increasing the risk of developing an infection [3]. Other factors such as psychological stress, lack of sleep and malnutrition can also depress immunity [4] and lead to increased risk of infection (fig. 1). There are also some situations in which an athlete's exposure to infectious agents may be increased, which is the other important determinant of infection risk. During exercise, exposure to airborne bacteria and viruses increases because of the higher rate and depth of breathing. An increase in gut permeability may also allow entry of gut bacterial endotoxins into the circulation, particularly during prolonged exercise in the heat. In contact sports skin abrasions may occur increasing the risk of transdermal infections. In some sports, the competitors may be in close proximity to large crowds. Air travel to foreign countries may be involved. Hence, the cause of the increased incidence of infection in athletes is most likely multifactorial (fig. 1). A variety of stressors (physical, psychological, environmental, and nutritional) suppress immune function, and these effects, together with increased exposure to potentially disease-causing pathogens, make the athlete more susceptible to infection.

Maintaining an Effective Immune System

Adequate nutrition and in particular appropriate intakes of energy, protein, vitamins and minerals are essential to maintain the body's natural defenses against disease-causing viruses and bacteria. Athletes are best advised to consume a sound diet that meets their energy needs and contains a variety of foods as the key to maintaining an effective immune system is to avoid deficiencies of the nutrients that play an essential role in immune cell functions [5]. Inadequate protein-energy intake or deficiencies of certain micronutrients (e.g. iron, zinc, magnesium, manganese, selenium, copper and vitamins A, C, D, E, B_6, B_{12} and folic acid) decrease immune defenses against invading pathogens and make the individual more susceptible to infection [5]. Even short-term dieting in athletes who continue to train hard that results in a loss of a few kilograms body mass over the course of a few weeks can result in significant falls in several aspects of immune function. Thus, care should be taken to ensure adequate protein (and micronutrient) intakes during periods of intentional weight loss, and it should be recognized that athletes undergoing weight reduction are likely to be more prone to infection. In general, a broad-range multivitamin/mineral supplement is the best choice to support a restricted food intake, and this may also be suitable for the travelling athlete in situations where food choices and quality may be limited. It has only recently been recognized that vitamin D plays an important role in upregulating immunity [6], and this is a concern as vitamin D insufficiency is common in athletes [7], especially if exposure to natural sunlight is limited (e.g. when training in the winter months or when training mostly indoors). An increasing number of studies in athletes and the general population have provided evidence that sufficient vitamin D status optimizes immune function and helps defend against the common cold. Hence, athletes who are deficient or insufficient in vitamin D (this can be established with a blood test to measure the circulating concentration of 25-hydroxy-vitamin D) are likely to benefit from vitamin D supplementation. For further details see the chapter on 'vitamin D supplementation in athletes' by Enette Larson-Meyer [pp. 109–121].

Nutrition Strategies to Limit Exercise-Induced Immune Depression

Certain supplements may boost immune function and reduce infection risk in individuals who are subjected to stress [5]. While there are many nutritional supplements on the market that are claimed to boost immunity (table 1), such claims are often based on selective evidence of efficacy in animals, in vitro experiments,

Table 1. Immune-boosting supplements – claims and the scientific evidence for efficacy in humans

Arginine	yyyyy	Nonessential amino acid that is a precursor in the synthesis of nitric oxide which is a cytotoxic molecule capable of destroying microorganisms and virus-infected cells. Claimed to enhance immune response and increase resistance to infection. There is no evidence that arginine has any effect on immunity in healthy humans.
β-Glucan	llyyy	A polysaccharide derived from the cell wall of yeast, fungi, algae, and oats that stimulates immunity. Oral feedings of oat β-glucan can offset exercise-induced immune suppression and decrease susceptibility to URTI in mice exercising heavily for 3 days. No evidence yet of a similar benefit for human athletes.
Bovine colostrum	lyyyy	First milk of the cow that contains antibodies, growth factors and cytokines. Claimed to boost mucosal immunity and increase resistance to infection. One study suggests an effect in elevating salivary IgA in human endurance runners but no evidence that this modifies infection risk.
Carbohydrate	lllyy	Ingestion of carbohydrate (30–60 g/h) attenuates stress hormone and (some) immune perturbations during exercise but only very limited evidence that this modifies infection risk in human athletes.
Curcumin	yyyyy	A component of the Indian spice turmeric and has potent anti-inflammatory activity. There is no evidence that curcumin has any effect on immunity in healthy humans.
Echinacea	yyyyy	Herbal extract that is a popular supplement among athletes. Claimed to boost immunity via stimulatory effects on macrophages. Early human studies indicated possible beneficial effects, but more recent, larger scale and better controlled studies indicate no effect of Echinacea on infection incidence or cold symptom severity.
Ginseng (Asian or Panax)	yyyyy	Asian ginseng (*Panax ginseng*) has been a part of Chinese medicine for over 2,000 years and was traditionally used to improve mental and physical vitality. Evidence for immune-modulating effects in humans is lacking.
Probiotics	lllyy	Probiotics are live microorganisms which when administered orally for several weeks, can increase the numbers of beneficial bacteria in the gut and modulate systemic immune function. Some placebo-controlled studies in athletes have indicated that daily probiotic ingestion results in fewer days of respiratory illness and lower severity of symptoms but larger scale studies are needed.
Plant polyphenols	llyyy	Quercetin is a flavonol (polyphenol) compound found in onions, apples, red wine, broccoli, tea, and Ginkgo biloba. It has antioxidant activities, inhibits protein kinases and regulates gene expression. Some limited evidence of reduced infection risk in human athletes with quercetin but mechanism of action unclear. A study with a NAB polyphenol beverage showed reduced inflammation and respiratory infection incidence after a marathon.
Vitamin C	llyyy	An essential water-soluble antioxidant vitamin taken in megadoses by many athletes. Some evidence from some (but not all) human studies that high-dose vitamin C (>200 mg/day) can be effective in reducing infection risk in stress situations and following ultramarathon races. May work by reducing stress hormone and anti-inflammatory cytokine responses to exercise.

Table 1. Continued

Vitamin D	lllyy	An essential fat-soluble vitamin that is known to have immunomodulatory effects. An increasing number of studies in athletes and the general population indicate that sufficient vitamin D status optimizes immune function and defends against respiratory infections. Thus, athletes who have deficient or insufficient vitamin D status are likely to benefit from supplementation.
Vitamin E	lyyyy	An essential fat-soluble antioxidant vitamin that is another popular supplement taken in megadoses by athletes. Good evidence for some immune-boosting effects in the frail elderly, but no evidence of similar benefit for younger healthy humans or athletes.
Zinc	lyyyy	An essential mineral that is claimed to reduce incidence and duration of colds. No evidence for reduced infection incidence with zinc supplementation in adult humans. Some (but not all) human studies suggest a reduction in duration of cold symptoms if zinc gluconate lozenges are administered within 24 h of cold symptom onset. Unlikely to be of any real benefit to athletes unless they are zinc deficient.

The scientific evidence is indicated with lllll meaning very strong evidence and yyyyy meaning limited to no evidence.

children, the elderly or clinical patients in severe catabolic states, and direct evidence for their efficacy for preventing exercise-induced immune depression or improving immune system status in athletes is usually lacking. The bulk of this short review focuses on describing the limited number of nutritional strategies and supplements for which there is some supportive scientific evidence base for efficacy in reducing immune perturbations during exercise and/or in decreasing infection incidence.

Carbohydrate Beverages

Carbohydrate ingestion during exercise limits metabolic stress by helping to maintain the blood glucose concentration. The use of a high-carbohydrate diet and carbohydrate ingestion (about 30–60 g/h) during prolonged workouts lowers circulating stress hormone (e.g. adrenaline and cortisol) and anti-inflammatory cytokine (e.g. interleukins 6 and 10) responses to exercise and delays the appearance of symptoms of overreaching during intensive training periods [8]. This reduces the impact of prolonged exercise on several, but not all, aspects of immune function, although evidence is currently lacking to demonstrate that this translates to a reduced incidence of illness symptoms following competitive events. When training sessions are performed in a fasting or low-glycogen state and without carbohydrate ingestion during exercise, it is likely that a more substantial degree of immune depression will develop (especially if this is not the first training session of the day).

If this train-low (glycogen) concept is to be applied to maximize training adaptation [9], it should not be done for more than a few days per week or immune function will be compromised.

The consumption of beverages during exercise not only helps prevent dehydration (which is associated with an increased stress hormone response) but also helps to maintain saliva flow rate during exercise. Saliva contains several proteins with antimicrobial properties including immunoglobulin A, lysozyme and α-amylase. Saliva secretion usually falls during exercise, but regular fluid intake during exercise can prevent this.

Antioxidant Vitamins

Although it is not known whether hard training increases the need for dietary antioxidants – as the body naturally develops an effective defense with a balanced diet and endogenous antioxidant defenses actually improve with exercise training – some recent evidence suggests that regular intake of relatively high doses of antioxidant vitamins can also reduce the stress response to prolonged exercise [10, 11]. These studies have used combinations of vitamin C and E, or vitamin C alone, and provide a possible mechanism to explain earlier findings of a benefit of vitamin C supplementation in reducing the incidence of respiratory illness symptoms in individuals who took part in ultramarathon races [12].

The most recent Cochrane meta-analysis examined the evidence that daily doses of more than 200 mg vitamin C were more effective in preventing or treating the common cold than placebo [13]. Twenty-nine trial comparisons involving 11,077 study participants contributed to this meta-analysis on the relative risk (RR) of developing a cold while taking prophylactic vitamin C. The pooled RR was 0.96 (95% CI: 0.92–1.00). A subgroup of six trials that involved physically active subjects (a total of 642 marathon runners, skiers, and soldiers on sub-arctic exercises) reported a pooled RR of 0.50 (95% CI: 0.38–0.66). Thirty comparisons that involved 9,676 respiratory episodes contributed to the meta-analysis on common cold duration during vitamin C or placebo supplementation. A consistent benefit of vitamin C was observed, representing a reduction in cold duration of 8% (95% CI: 3–13%) for adult participants. Fifteen trial comparisons that involved 7,045 respiratory episodes contributed to the meta-analysis of severity of episodes, and the results revealed a benefit of vitamin C when days confined to home and off work or school were taken as a measure of severity. The authors concluded that the failure of vitamin C supplementation to reduce the incidence of colds in the normal population indicates that routine ingestion of mega-doses of vitamin C is not generally justified but that individuals subjected to periods of severe physical exercise and/or cold environments may well gain some benefit. However, even if some protective effect of high-dose antioxidant supplementation on infection risk is indeed a reality, athletes need to consider the risks that may include the blunting of some of the adaptations to training with a high intake of antioxidants [14], though whether or not this is likely to affect adaptations in already well-trained athletes performing intensive training has recently been questioned [15]. Excessive supplementation with other antioxidant vitamins cannot be recommended because there is little evidence of benefit, while it is known that oversupplementation can actually diminish the body's natural antioxidant defense system. Ensuring that the diet contains plenty of fresh fruits and vegetables is probably the wisest option.

Immunonutrition Support for Athletes

Various other nutritional supplements have been tested for their capacity to reduce immune changes following prolonged strenuous exercise and thus lower infection risk. This strategy is similar to the immunonutrition support provided to patients recovering from trauma and surgery, and to the frail elderly. Supplements studied thus far in human athletes include zinc, omega-3 polyunsaturated fatty acids, herbal extracts (e.g. Echinacea), plant sterols, polyphenols (e.g. quercetin) and polysaccharides (e.g. β-glucan), glutamine, branched-chain amino acids, and bovine colostrum. Although some supplements (e.g. zinc [16] and some herbals such as Kaloba [17]) may reduce severity or duration of illness if taken close to the onset of symptoms, thus far results have been generally disappointing with regard to reducing infection incidence (see table 1), and focus has shifted to examining the effects of probiotics and plant polyphenols.

Plant Polyphenols
Plant polyphenols are potent antioxidant compounds. One of these, quercetin, has received a lot of attention in recent years in relation to its possible effects on exercise performance, training adaptation and immune function. Quercetin is classified as a flavonoid, a phytonutrient found in a variety of fruits and vegetables. The physiologic effects of these compounds are of great current interest due to their antioxidant, anti-inflammatory, antipathogenic, cardioprotective, and anticarcinogenic activities. Animal studies indicate that 7 days of quercetin feeding improves survival from influenza virus inoculation. A recent human study [18] showed that 1,000 mg of a quercetin supplement ingested daily for 3 weeks significantly increased plasma quercetin levels and reduced respiratory illness during the 2 weeks following a 3-day period of exhaustive exercise in cyclists. Immune dysfunction, inflammation, and oxidative stress, however, were not altered, suggesting that quercetin may have exerted direct antiviral effects. Another study

reported a lower incidence of respiratory infections among physically active middle-aged people with daily quercetin supplementation [19], but larger scale, double-blind, placebo-controlled studies are needed to confirm an effect of quercetin in reducing infection incidence in athletes who are training hard. Naturally occurring polyphenolic compounds are present in foods such green leafy vegetables, onions, apples, pears, citrus fruits and red grapes as well as some plant-based beverages such as citrus juices, green tea, red wine and beer. A recent study investigated whether regular ingestion of non-alcoholic beer (NAB) polyphenols prior to and after a marathon would attenuate post-race inflammation and decrease the incidence of respiratory illness symptoms [20]. Healthy middle-aged male runners (n = 277) were randomly assigned to drink 1–1.5 l per day of a NAB or placebo beverage for 3 weeks before and 2 weeks after a marathon race. Blood markers of inflammation were significantly reduced in NAB compared to placebo immediately after the race and 24 h later and the incidence of respiratory illness was 3.25-fold lower in the NAB group compared with the placebo group during the 2-week post-marathon period. Another recent study that examined the effects of regular ingestion of dark chocolate (cocoa is another source of polyphenols) prior to an exhausting bout of cycling reported reduced oxidative stress markers but no effects on hormonal or immune responses to the exercise [21], so the type and dose of polyphenols may be important.

Probiotics

In recent years, several studies have examined the efficacy of oral probiotics in athletes, and some of these, particularly those containing *Lactobacillus* strains, have shown some promise. Often called the friendly bacteria, probiotics are live microorganisms which when administered in adequate amounts, modify the bacterial population that inhabits our gut and modulate immune function by their interaction with the gut-associated lymphoid tissue, leading to positive effects on the systemic immune system. Some well-controlled studies in athletes have indicated that daily probiotic ingestion results in fewer days of respiratory illness and lower severity of upper respiratory tract infection (URTI) symptoms [22–25], and a recent meta-analysis using data from both athlete and non-athlete studies involving 3,451 subjects concluded that there is a likely benefit in reducing URTI incidence [26]. Thus, probiotic supplements may convey some benefit to immunity and reduce URTI incidence as well as reduce gastrointestinal problems (a common complaint of endurance runners). Another potential benefit of probiotics could be a reduced risk of gastrointestinal infections – a particular concern when travelling abroad. Further large-scale studies are needed to confirm that taking probiotics can reduce the number of training days lost to infection and to determine the most effective probiotics as their effects are strain specific. The studies to date that have shown reduced URTI incidence in athletes have been mostly limited to *Lactobacillus* species and have used daily doses of ~10^{10} live bacteria. Given that some probiotics appear to provide some benefit with no evidence of harm and are low cost, there is no reason why athletes should not take probiotics, especially if travelling abroad or illness prone.

Colostrum
Bovine colostrum is the first collection of a thick creamy-yellow liquid, produced by the mammary gland of a lactating cow shortly after birth of her calf, usually within the first 36 h. Colostrum contains antibodies, growth factors, enzymes, gangliosides (acid glycosphingolipids), vitamins and minerals, and is commercially available in both liquid and powder forms. Numerous health claims have been made for colostrum ranging from performance enhancement to preventing infections, but well-controlled studies in athletes are rare. The gangliosides in colostrum may modify the gut microbial flora and act as decoy targets for bacterial adhesion as well as having some direct immunostimulatory properties. A few studies suggest that several weeks of bovine colostrum supplementation can elevate levels of antibodies in the circulation and saliva, prevent exercise-induced falls in salivary lysozyme and speed the recovery of neutrophil function after strenuous exercise [27, 28]. Further studies are needed to confirm and extend these observations of effects on immune responses to exercise and to establish if bovine colostrum can reduce the incidence of URTIs in athletes.

Conclusions

It is difficult to make firm judgments about which nutritional supplements are really effective in boosting immunity or reducing infection risk in athletes. It is safe to say with reasonable confidence that individual amino acids, colostrum, Echinacea, vitamin E and zinc are unlikely to be of benefit. The ingestion of adequate amounts of protein and micronutrients in the diet (vitamin D status may be of particular concern), intake of carbohydrate during exercise and daily consumption of probiotic and plant polyphenol (e.g. quercetin) supplements currently offer the best chance of success. This approach is likely to be most effective in those individuals who are particularly prone to illness. Athletes might consider taking zinc and Kaloba supplements in the days leading up to an important competition just in case they do come down with a cold at that important time. It is important to remember that nutrition is only one factor with regard to infection risk, and there are several other strategies listed below that can minimize the risk of developing immune function depression or reduce the degree of exposure to pathogens and thus limit infection risk.

Minimize the chances of developing immunodepression:
- Avoid very prolonged training sessions (>2 h), overtraining and chronic fatigue
- Keep other life stresses to a minimum
- Get adequate sleep quantity (at least 7 h) and quality
- Avoid rapid weight loss
- Vaccinate against influenza if competing in the winter

Minimize the potential for transmission of infectious agents:
- Avoid sick people and large crowds in enclosed spaces if possible
- Good personal skin and oral hygiene (wash hands and use antimicrobial gels on hands; brush teeth regularly and use an antibacterial mouth rinse)
- Never share drink bottles, cutlery, towels, etc.
- Avoid putting hands to eyes and nose (a major route of viral self-inoculation)

Disclosure Statement

The author has received funding for research from GlaxoSmithKline, Nestlé and Yakult.

References

1. Gleeson M (ed): Immune Function in Sport and Exercise. Edinburgh, Elsevier, 2005.
2. Bermon S: Airway inflammation and upper respiratory tract infection in athletes: is there a link? Exerc Immunol Rev 2007;13:6–14.
3. Walsh NP, Gleeson M, Shephard RJ, et al: Position statement part one: immune function and exercise. Exerc Immunol Rev 2011;17:6–63.
4. Walsh NP, Gleeson M, Pyne DB, et al: Position statement part two: maintaining immune health. Exerc Immunol Rev 2011;17:64–103.
5. Gleeson M: Exercise, nutrition and immunity; in Calder PC, Yaqoob P (eds): Diet, Immunity and Inflammation. Cambridge, Woodhead Publishing, 2012, chapter 30.
6. Kamen DL, Tangpricha V: Vitamin D and molecular actions on the immune system: modulation of innate and autoimmunity. J Mol Med 2010;88:441–450.
7. Larson-Meyer DE, Willis KS: Vitamin D and athletes. Curr Sports Med Rep 2010;9:220–226.
8. Halson SL, Lancaster GI, Achten J, et al: Effect of carbohydrate supplementation on performance and carbohydrate oxidation following intensified cycling training. J Appl Physiol 2004;97:1245–1253.
9. Hawley JA, Burke LM: Carbohydrate availability and training adaptation: effects on cell metabolism. Exerc Sport Sci Rev 2010;38:152–160.
10. Fischer CP, Hiscock NJ, Penkowa M, et al: Supplementation with vitamins C and E inhibits the release of interleukin-6 from contracting human skeletal muscle. J Physiol 2004;558:633–645.
11. Davison G, Gleeson M: The effect of 2 weeks vitamin C supplementation on immunoendocrine responses to 2.5 h cycling exercise in man. Eur J Appl Physiol 2006;97:454–461.

12 Peters EM: Vitamins, immunity, and infection risk in athletes; in Nieman DC, Pedersen BK (eds): Nutrition and Exercise Immunology. Boca Raton, CRC Press, 2000, pp 109–136.
13 Douglas RM, Hemila H, Chalker E, et al: Vitamin C for preventing and treating the common cold. Cochrane Database Syst Rev 2007;CD000980.
14 Ristow M, Zarse K, Oberbach A, et al: Antioxidants prevent health-promoting effects of physical exercise in humans. Proc Natl Acad Sci 2009;106:8665–8670.
15 Yfanti C, Akerström T, Nielsen S, et al: Antioxidant supplementation does not alter endurance training adaptation. Med Sci Sports Exerc 2010;42:1388–1395.
16 Singh M, Das RR: Zinc for the common cold. Cochrane Database Syst Rev 2011;CD001364.
17 Timmer A, Gunther J, Rucker G, et al: *Pelargonium sidoides* extract for acute respiratory tract infections. Cochrane Database Syst Rev 2008;CD006323.
18 Nieman DC, Henson DA, Gross SJ, et al: Quercetin reduces illness but not immune perturbations after intensive exercise. Med Sci Sports Exerc 2007;39:1561–1569.
19 Heinz SA, Henson DA, Austin MD, et al: Quercetin supplementation and upper respiratory tract infection: a randomized community clinical trial. Pharmacol Res 2010;62:237–242.
20 Scherr J, Nieman DC, Schuster T, et al: Nonalcoholic beer reduces inflammation and incidence of respiratory tract illness. Med Sci Sports Exerc 2012;44:18–26.
21 Allgrove JE, Farrell E, Gleeson M, et al: Regular dark chocolate consumption's reduction of oxidative stress and increase of free-fatty-acid mobilization in response to prolonged cycling. Int J Sport Nutr Exerc Metab 2011;21:113–123.
22 Gleeson M, Thomas L: Exercise and immune function. Is there any evidence for probiotic benefit for sports people? Comp Nutr 2008;8:35–37.
23 Cox AJ, Pyne DB, Saunders PU, et al: Oral administration of the probiotic *Lactobacillus fermentum* VRI-003 and mucosal immunity in endurance athletes. Br J Sports Med 2010;44:222–226.
24 Gleeson M, Bishop NC, Oliveira M, et al: Daily probiotic's (*Lactobacillus casei* Shirota) reduction of infection incidence in athletes. Int J Sport Nutr Exerc Metab 2011;21:55–64.
25 West NP, Pyne DB, Cripps AW, et al: *Lactobacillus fermentum* (PCC(R)) supplementation and gastrointestinal and respiratory-tract illness symptoms: a randomised control trial in athletes. Nutr J 2011;10:30.
26 Hao Q, Lu Z, Dong BR, et al: Probiotics for preventing acute upper respiratory tract infections. Cochrane Database Syst Rev 2011;CD006895.
27 Crooks CV, Wall CR, Cross ML, et al: The effect of bovine colostrum supplementation on salivary IgA in distance runners. Int J Sport Nutr Exerc Metabol 2006;16:47–64.
28 Davison G, Diment BC: Bovine colostrum supplementation attenuates the decrease of salivary lysozyme and enhances the recovery of neutrophil function after prolonged exercise. Br J Nutr 2010;103:1425–1432.

Questions and Answers

Question 1: Vitamins are important to maintain proper immune function, and many athletes are taking vitamin supplements. Would you recommend using vitamin supplements?

Answer: Yes, I would. Vitamins are essential for the normal functioning of the immune system. If you become deficient in virtually any of them, but particularly vitamin A, vitamin E, vitamin B_{12} or folic acid, your immune system actually goes down, and it won't function as well, and you're more likely to get infections. One way of protecting against that is to simply take a multivitamin tablet on a daily basis. So yes, I would recommend them.

Question 2: What actually causes infections?

Answer: Infections are caused mostly by viruses. The most common infection that athletes and the general population get is the common cold, and 90% of common colds are caused by viruses. The other 10% or so are the result of bacterial infections.

Question 3: Is it true that endurance athletes like cyclists get more infections than weightlifters, for example?

Answer: In general, yes. The endurance athletes get more infections than the power athletes and the sprinters. This is thought to be because the long hard hours of training that the endurance athletes do actually cause sufficient stress to depress their immunity, at least temporarily for several hours after exercise. In fact, there have been some studies done where people have run a marathon, and the guys who have run the marathon actually come down with more infections in the week or two afterwards compared to guys that might have trained for the marathon but didn't compete for reasons other than illness.

Question 4: Are there any nutritional strategies to minimize the risk of infections for endurance athletes?

Answer: There's only a few that we can currently recommend because the evidence isn't very clear on a lot of things. There are so many of those things in the health food shops that are claimed to boost immunity, but most of the studies that have been done in athletes have shown that they don't really work. Of the things that do work, we know, the most important is to avoid deficiencies of energy, protein and all the essential micronutrients you need. Not only vitamins, but also minerals like manganese, iron and zinc, are very important for maintaining immunity. Taking probiotics is probably a good idea. There have been a number of recent studies using the *Lactobacillus* species of probiotics that show a positive effect in reducing infection incidence and in some cases also reducing the severity or duration of infections when they do occur in endurance athletes.

Question 5: What about additional antioxidants?

Answer: That's a difficult one to answer. There were some studies done in the 1990s by Edith Peter's group in South Africa. They reported that taking high doses of vitamin C in particular for several weeks before running an ultra-marathon race decreased the incidence of infections when compared with a placebo treatment. But subsequently, in recent years the story has come about that if you take high doses of antioxidant vitamins, it might actually impair some of the adaptations to training. This is because when we do exercise, we generate some increased free radicals or reactive oxygen species, and these are thought to be important signals in the training adaptation process. So, taking too high levels of antioxidant vitamins might actually quench those free radicals as they're being produced and so prevent or limit the training adaptations. However, those studies have actually mostly been done either in animals or untrained humans. There are one or two more recent studies that are coming out now that have looked at already well-trained athletes. When these guys take high doses of combined vitamins C and vitamin E for several months, no performance changes, and no impairment to training adaptations has been reported in those studies. So it's not really clear whether or not they do have a negative effect. Athletes take high-dose vitamin C because they've probably heard or read something that tells them that it might reduce their risk of infection, and that was really based on the studies that were done in the 1990s. We now know that one of the mechanisms by which the antioxidants might be working actually is by suppressing cortisol release during exercise. Cortisol is a stress hormone that depresses immunity. So, if you can prevent that being secreted or reduce its secretion, you don't get as much immune depression with your exercise bout.

Question 6: Do you believe that a lot of athletes are having micronutrient deficiency?

Answer: Well, that seems to be so certainly when these nutrition surveys are done or when you test the blood of athletes to see what their vitamin status is, for example. A number of studies show that iron status is usually a little bit on the low side. So they have low levels of serum ferritin and possibly low levels of hemoglobin, which would actually impair performance. You certainly don't want that. But vitamin D is another one that has come up recently. It has been recognized in the last 3 or 4 years that vitamin D is actually very important for maintaining normal immune function. It actually stimulates the activity of some of our immune cells. Some studies indicate that vitamin D insufficiency is quite common among athletes.

Question 7: And what about vitamins C or E?

Answer: These vitamins are rarely deficient. We usually get enough of those in the diet, provided that you are eating plenty of fruit and vegetables. That's probably the best way to get the vitamins and minerals you need.

Use of β-Alanine as an Ergogenic Aid

Wim Derave

Department of Movement and Sports Sciences, Ghent University, Ghent, Belgium

Abstract

Despite the large variety of so-called ergogenic supplements used by the sporting community, only few of them are effectively supported by scientific proof. One of the recent evidence-based supplements that entered the market is β-alanine. β-Alanine is the rate-limiting precursor for the synthesis of the dipeptide carnosine (β-alanyl-L-histidine) in human muscle. The chronic daily ingestion of β-alanine can markedly elevate muscle carnosine content, which results in improved exercise capacity, especially in sports that include high-intensity exercise episodes. The use of β-alanine is exponentially growing in recent years. This chapter aims to (1) discuss the scientific basis and physiological background of β-alanine and its synthesis product carnosine, and (2) translate these scientific findings to practical applications in sports.

Copyright © 2013 Nestec Ltd., Vevey/S. Karger AG, Basel

Muscle Carnosine Loading by β-Alanine Supplementation

The successful development of a new dietary supplement for sports often depends on identifying a molecule (usually in muscle) which has a critical and limiting role in the energy delivery system during exercise and which can be influenced (usually elevated) by nutritional intervention. A number of scientific discovery steps (see table 1) need to be established before a new supplement is ready for evidence-based application in sports. The rational development of β-alanine as an ergogenic supplement has been established mainly by Roger Harris and coworkers over the last decade. The discovery steps for β-alanine are explained in table 1. For a full description of the story of its discovery, we refer to more extensive recent review papers [1, 2].

Table 1. Stepwise discovery and scientific support for the use of β-alanine as a sport supplement

	Questions to be answered during the development steps	Answers for carnosine/β-alanine	Reference
1	Is there a good rationale? Is the molecule critical for performance?	1. Carnosine has good pH buffering capacity and other beneficial biochemical properties 2. Strong evolutionary drive for carnosine content in muscle of animals with high anaerobic energy delivery system (racing dogs and horses)	[20]
2	Is the molecule (or its precursor) readily absorbed in the gut?	Good intestinal absorption of β-alanine and carnosine	[5]
3	Are there no major side effects?	Only paresthesia occurs when β-alanine ingestion exceeds 10 mg/kg bodyweight. No other side effects reported so far.	[5]
4	Which nutritional intervention is able to elevate the molecule content in skeletal muscle?	1. β-Alanine was identified as the rate-limiting precursor for the synthesis of carnosine in muscle 2. Carnosine is elevated in muscle by 50–80% by ingesting 4–6 g/day of β-alanine during 4–10 consecutive weeks	[5, 12]
5	Is the nutritional intervention also able to elevate the molecule content in muscle of trained athletes (who usually already have an optimized system)?	Carnosine is elevated by 40% in muscle of well-trained runners	[9]
6	In which exercise types does an elevated muscle content indeed lead to improved performance?	A pronounced ergogenic effect of chronic β-alanine ingestion was found for a high-intensity exercise capacity test (cycling at 110% of W_{max}) lasting approx. 2.5 min	[12]

In short, carnosine (β-alanyl-L-histidine) is a dipeptide synthesized from the precursors β-alanine and L-histidine [3]. It was discovered in 1900 as one of the first identified molecules in meat extract. Carnosine is present in high concentrations in skeletal muscle of humans (~5–8 mmol/l wet muscle or ~20–30 mmol/kg dry muscle) and other vertebrates. It is evident that a molecule with such a high concentration in muscle must have an important role in homeostasis and/or energy delivery during exercise. Consequently, one would expect that a method that would elevate the content of carnosine in muscle, will lead to improved exercise capacity, at least in some exercise types. More than a century after its discovery, Harris and co-workers were the first to demonstrate that chronic β-alanine supplementation is effective in elevating intramuscular carnosine concentration, first in horses [4] and later in humans [5]. Thus β-alanine, and not histidine, is the rate-limiting precursor for carnosine synthesis. It would also be possible to ingest carnosine itself as a food supplement. However, the manufacturing costs of carnosine are much higher than for β-alanine. Therefore, the latter had more economical potential.

There are a number of typical characteristics of β-alanine supplementation in relation to muscle carnosine loading which have now been identified, and which will have implications for its use in sports.

Almost Everyone Is a Responder
In contrast to other supplements, such as creatine, the ability of β-alanine to elevate the muscle carnosine content is present in nearly all subjects. In our laboratory [6–9], several dozens of subjects have been supplemented with 4–5 g/day β-alanine for 4–6 weeks, and only one subject was found not to respond.

There Is No Ceiling Effect (Yet)
With creatine supplementation, subjects with an already high initial muscle creatine content showed little or no further increase upon supplementation, which is termed a ceiling effect. With β-alanine, no such effect has been found. Initial muscle carnosine content does not affect the degree of further increase upon β-alanine supplementation. Equally, the maximal attainable level of muscle carnosine content upon prolonged supplementation has not been determined yet.

Total Amount of Consumed β-Alanine Is the Major Determinant for Carnosine Loading
Stellingwerff et al. [10] recently showed that if you take a lower daily dose (1.6 g), it takes twice as long to load muscle carnosine to the same level as with a higher dose (3.2 g). Taking together several supplementation studies, it seems that the total amount of ingested β-alanine is the most decisive aspect of effective supplementation. A total amount of 100–200 g of β-alanine ingested over several weeks is expected to raise muscle carnosine content by 30–50%.

Carnosine Loading and Washout Are Slow
With an advised maximum daily dose of around 5 g/day, a supplementation period of 20–40 days is advisable to raise muscle carnosine content by 30–50% (see above). This means that one should optimally start supplement-

ing at least one month before an important competition to obtain optimal results. Likewise, the washout (the disappearance of carnosine from the muscle upon termination of a supplementation period) is slow, and may last 9 or more weeks before carnosine returns to pre-supplementation level [6, 10].

Slow-Release β-Alanine Avoids Side Effects
A commonly reported side effect of β-alanine supplements is a prickling and sometimes painful sensation of the skin of hands and face, called paresthesia. The cause of this side effect is not fully understood. However, it seems that the occurrence of paresthesia is avoided when ingesting small doses at once (not more than 10 mg/kg bodyweight, with 2-hour intervals) and even better by ingesting β-alanine in a slow-release formulation. The latter procedure avoids high circulating β-alanine levels and the concomitant paresthesia symptoms [11].

Use of β-Alanine in Various Exercise Types and Sport Disciplines

The first evidence for the ergogenic potential of β-alanine came from Hill et al. [12], who demonstrated that β-alanine supplementation can improve high-intensity exercise capacity by 13–16% during a cycle capacity test at 110% of the maximal power output following 4 and 10 weeks' supplementation. Since then, over 20 studies have explored β-alanine's effects in a number of exercise types and target populations. A good meta-analysis of the performance results of these studies has recently been provided by Hobson et al. [13]. The meta-analysis was performed on 57 effect sizes on a total of 360 subjects. It distinguished three types of exercise: (1) exercises which lasted <60 s, (2) efforts between 60 and 240 s, and (3) efforts longer than 240 s. It can be concluded that efforts which lasted less than 60 s are unlikely to benefit from β-alanine supplementation. In contrast, mainly the studies on exercise durations of 60–240 s showed a significantly higher effect size in the β-alanine versus the placebo groups. However, once exercise duration increased over 240 s, the beneficial effects of β-alanine supplementation became less pronounced, although still significant (table 2).

Although a number of studies have shown an ergogenic effect on single exercise bouts (summarized in Derave et al. [2]), there is only a limited availability of studies investigating the effect of β-alanine supplementation on repeated sprint ability. Derave et al. [9] showed that the fatigue during 5 bouts of 30 maximal knee extension contractions, separated by a 1-min passive recovery period,

Table 2. Results from the meta-analysis by Hobson et al. [13] on the effects of β-alanine vs. placebo supplementation on performance measures during exercise of varying durations

Exercise duration	Placebo average	range	β-Alanine average	range	p value
Shorter than 60 s	0.118	−0.037 to 0.471	0.193	0.072 to 0.540	0.312
60–240 s	0.121	0.087 to 0.221	0.665	0.481 to 1.110	0.001
Longer than 240 s	0.095	−0.059 to 0.607	0.368	0.133 to 0.797	0.046

was attenuated in the 4th and 5th bout following muscle carnosine loading. On the other hand, Sweeney et al. [14] could not demonstrate performance enhancement during repeated sprint exercise (10 × 5 s) following 5 weeks of β-alanine supplementation.

Ergogenic Mechanism of β-Alanine

It is a common misunderstanding that β-alanine is a pH buffer. β-Alanine itself has no buffering capacity. However, β-alanine is the rate-limiting precursor in the synthesis of carnosine, a dipeptide composed of histidine and β-alanine. Only histidine (especially when bound to β-alanine) is able to accept protons and act as a pH buffer. β-alanine ingestion is an effective way to increase the amount of carnosine in skeletal muscle and thereby indirectly increase the buffering capacity of a muscle.

Even though the contribution of carnosine to the total buffering capacity of the muscle in particular and the body in general, is rather small, there is a considerable interest in muscle carnosine because its concentration can be nutritionally altered. A recent study by Baguet et al. [8] showed that the acidosis during a 6-min high-intensity exercise bout is less pronounced as a result of a 4-week β-alanine supplementation period (fig. 1). This indicates that β-alanine-induced muscle carnosine loading has a significant impact on the pH buffering capacity during exercise.

Apart from the pH buffering capacity, carnosine possesses other properties that may contribute to performance enhancement. Interestingly, carnosine can promote both the release and sensitivity of calcium in the excitation-contraction mechanism, which has recently been shown in human muscle fibers [15] after previous evidence from animal muscles [16]. Additionally, carnosine could be functioning as an antioxidant, and thereby antagonize muscle fatigue, although the evidence for the latter mechanism is very scarce

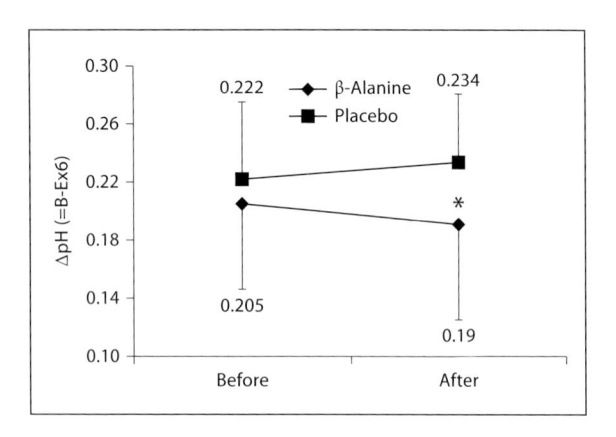

Fig. 1. ΔpH from baseline to the end (6 min) of high-intensity cycling before and after 4 weeks' supplementation of β-alanine or placebo. Data are mean ± SD of 7 subjects per group. * p = 0.03, significant interaction effect. Figure from Baguet et al. [8].

[17]. The precise mechanism(s) of carnosine's ergogenic effect needs further elucidation as this will allow us to better identify and predict the type of exercise and sports where the use of β-alanine is warranted.

Carnosine Loading and Bicarbonate Ingestion: Two Different Ways of Fighting Acidosis?

Intense contractions during high-intensity exercise result in large proton production, which leads to acidosis within skeletal muscle cells. A significant portion of the contraction-induced protons are rapidly transported out of the active muscles and buffered by the circulating buffers, such as bicarbonate. This state of acidosis in muscle and blood is presumably one of the causes of fatigue. Therefore, one could term the pH buffers inside the muscle cells (such as carnosine) as the *first line of defense* and the blood buffers as the *second line of defense* against high-intensity exercise fatigue.

A more established way to tackle the acidosis (through the second line of defense) is to start the exercise with a higher than normal blood pH, i.e. induced alkalosis. This can be achieved by pre-exercise ingestion of sodium bicarbonate in a dose of 0.18–0.3 g/kg bodyweight, or another alkalizing agent, such as sodium citrate. This strategy has proven to be successful in enhancing performance in single or repeated high-intensity exercise bouts. From the above, it is evident that nutritional support of both systems (muscle buffering through carnosine loading and blood buffering through bicarbonate inges-

Table 3. Comparison between the two most popular pH-buffering nutritional supplements

	Bicarbonate	β-Alanine
Physiological mechanism	Makes blood more alkaline (pH >7.4)	Increases the concentration of carnosine in skeletal muscle
Mode of administration	Acute single dose (0.18–0.3 g per kg bodyweight), 60–90 min prior to match	Chronic administration for 4–10 weeks (1.5–6 g/day) prior to and during match period
Duration of effects	1–3 h following ingestion	From 3–4 weeks following start of supplementation until 1 month following discontinuation
Makes blood more alkaline at rest	Yes	No
Attenuates acidosis during exercise	Yes	Yes
Evidence for ergogenic effects in single intense exercise bouts	Yes (duration 30 s to 7 min)	Yes (duration 60 s to 7 min)
Evidence for ergogenic effects in repeated maximal exercise bouts	Yes	Insufficient evidence currently available
Side effects	Gastrointestinal discomfort in some individuals, even at recommended dose	Temporary skin prickling (paresthesia) when exceeding the recommended dose (10 mg/kg bodyweight)

tion) can lead to performance-enhancing effects during intense exercise. Table 3 summarizes the similarities and differences between both supplements.

From table 3, it can be seen that bicarbonate and β-alanine each have their pros and cons, and that their modes of action are different. Consequently, it can be hypothesized that both effects are possibly additive. Sale et al. [18] have recently examined the time to exhaustion in a ~2.5-min intense exercise bout in subjects receiving both chronic β-alanine and acute sodium bicarbonate simultaneously. Another recent study by Bellinger et al. [19] explored the combined vs. single effects of β-alanine and bicarbonate in high-intensity cycling in well-trained athletes. The results of both studies are summarized in table 4. The data of both studies suggest that the highest and most consistent ergogenic effects are obtained when both supplement modes are combined. However, it must be mentioned that the researchers were not able to statistically support that the effect of combined supplementation was different from the effects of either supplement alone.

Table 4. Summary of two recent studies exploring the effects of β-alanine and bicarbonate supplementation, either combined or given alone, on high-intensity cycling performance

Reference	Performance test	Placebo	β-Alanine	Bicarbonate	β-Alanine + bicarbonate
[18]	Time to exhaustion at 110% W_{max} cycling	+1.6%	+12.1%*	+6.5%	+16.2%*
[19]	4-min maximal cycling performance trial	+0.3%	+1.45%	+3%*	+3.2%*

Asterix indicates significant improvement in performance compared to the pre-supplementation trial in the same subjects.

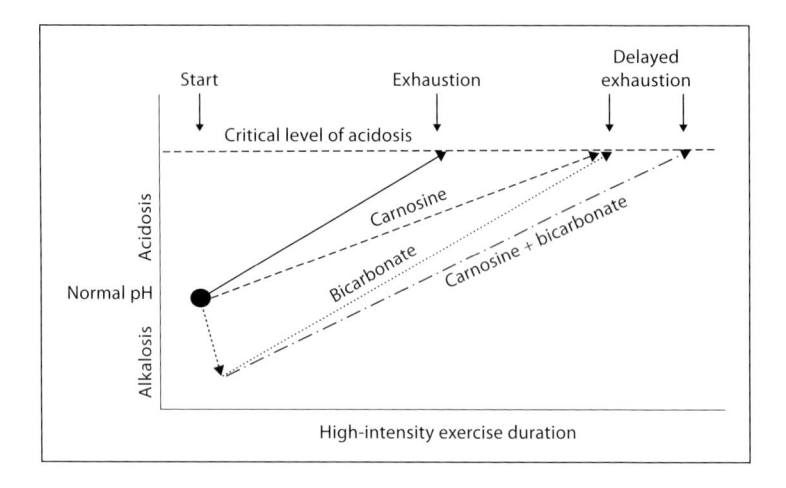

Fig. 2. Theoretical mechanism illustrating the effects and mechanisms of carnosine loading, bicarbonate ingestion and both interventions combined on the development of acidosis and fatigue during high-intensity exercise. For further explanations, see text.

Even though the actual evidence for an additive effect of β-alanine and bicarbonate is still modest at present, there is a theoretical framework which could explain this additivity. Figure 2 illustrates this framework. In high-intensity exercise, it is thought that exercise is stopped once the acidity of muscle and/or blood reaches a critical level of acidosis (horizontal dashed line). Theoretically, there are two ways to delay the time at which an exercising athlete reaches this point of exhaustion/fatigue. A first way is to start at a resting pH level which is further away from the critical acidosis level. This is accomplished by inducing metabolic alkalosis (i.e. the opposite of acidosis) by pre-exercise bicarbonate ingestion. This strategy could be compared with for example pre-exercise body cooling before exercising in the heat. If hyperthermia is a cause of fatigue when exercising in a hot climate, then pre-exercise hypothermia (cooling) is an effective way to delay the point of critical hyperthermia. It must be stressed that this strategy may have some drawbacks, because alkalosis itself (or hypothermia) may have side effects. A second way is to slow the speed of acid accumulation by providing a better muscular buffering system, which is met by β-alanine-induced carnosine loading. As both ways have different approaches, it could be possible to combine them and obtain an even better result than with either approach alone. As stated above, this has not been extensively tested at present, and the practical use in a sport setting may face additional limitations which are still unidentified.

Conclusions and Future Perspectives

It can be concluded that β-alanine can be added to the short list of evidence-based ergogenic supplements. The muscle carnosine loading in response to β-alanine supplementation seems to improve high-intensity exercise capacity, also in well-trained sportsmen.

Additional scientific exploration is required to further identify the ergogenic mechanism(s) and the range of sport applications. There is still a paucity of data on women and elite athletes, and on the effects and safety of long-term supplementation (several months). Finally, the interaction with other supplements needs further attention.

Disclosure Statement

The author declares no conflict of interest.

References

1 Sale C, Saunders B, Harris RC: Effect of beta-alanine supplementation on muscle carnosine concentrations and exercise performance. Amino Acids 2010;39:321–333.
2 Derave W, Everaert I, Beeckman S, Baguet A: Muscle carnosine metabolism and beta-alanine supplementation in relation to exercise and training. Sports Med 2010;40:247–263.
3 Boldyrev AA: Carnosine and Oxidative Stress in Cells and Tissues. New York, Nova Science Publishers, 2007.
4 Dunnett M, Harris RC: Influence of oral β-alanine and histidine supplementation on the carnosine content of the gluteus medius. Equine Vet J Suppl 1999;30:499–504.

5 Harris RC, Tallon MJ, Dunnett M, et al: The absorption of orally supplied beta-alanine and its effect on muscle carnosine synthesis in human vastus lateralis. Amino Acids 2006;30:279–289.

6 Baguet A, Reyngoudt H, Pottier A, et al: Carnosine loading and washout in human skeletal muscles. J Appl Physiol 2009;106:837–842.

7 Baguet A, Bourgois J, Vanhee L, et al: Important role of muscle carnosine in rowing performance. J Appl Physiol 2010;109:1096–1101.

8 Baguet A, Koppo K, Pottier A, Derave W: Beta-alanine supplementation reduces acidosis but not oxygen uptake response during high-intensity cycling exercise. Eur J Appl Physiol 2010;108:495–503.

9 Derave W, Ozdemir MS, Harris RC, et al: Beta-alanine supplementation augments muscle carnosine content and attenuates fatigue during repeated isokinetic contraction bouts in trained sprinters. J Appl Physiol 2007;103:1736–1743.

10 Stellingwerff T, Anwander H, Egger A, et al: Effect of two beta-alanine dosing protocols on muscle carnosine synthesis and washout. Amino Acids 2012;42:2461–2472.

11 Decombaz J, Beaumont M, Vuichoud J, et al: Effect of slow-release beta-alanine tablets on absorption kinetics and paresthesia. Amino Acids 2012;43:67–76.

12 Hill CA, Harris RC, Kim HJ, et al: Influence of beta-alanine supplementation on skeletal muscle carnosine concentrations and high intensity cycling capacity. Amino Acids 2007;32:225–233.

13 Hobson RM, Saunders B, Ball G, et al: Effects of beta-alanine supplementation on exercise performance: a meta-analysis. Amino Acids 2012;43:25–37.

14 Sweeney KM, Wright GA, Glenn BA, Doberstein ST: The effect of beta-alanine supplementation on power performance during repeated sprint activity. J Strength Cond Res 2010;24:79–87.

15 Dutka TL, Lamboley CR, Mckenna MJ, et al: Effects of carnosine on contractile apparatus Ca^{2+}-sensitivity and sarcoplasmic reticulum Ca^{2+} release in human skeletal muscle fibers. J Appl Physiol 2012;112:728–736.

16 Dutka TL, Lamb GD: Effect of carnosine on excitation-contraction coupling in mechanically-skinned rat skeletal muscle. J Muscle Res Cell Motil 2004;25:203–213.

17 Smith AE, Stout JR, Kendall KL, et al: Exercise-induced oxidative stress: the effects of beta-alanine supplementation in women. Amino Acids 2012;43:77–90.

18 Sale C, Saunders B, Hudson S, et al: Effect of beta-alanine plus sodium bicarbonate on high-intensity cycling capacity. Med Sci Sports Exerc 2011;43:1972–1978.

19 Bellinger PM, Howe ST, Shing CM, Fell JW: Effect of combined β-alanine and sodium bicarbonate supplementation on cycling performance. Med Sci Sports Exerc 2012;44:1545–1551.

20 Abe H: Role of histidine-related compounds as intracellular proton buffering constituents in vertebrate muscle. Biochemistry (Mosc) 2000;65:757–765.

Vitamin D Supplementation in Athletes

Enette Larson-Meyer

University of Wyoming, Laramie, WY, USA

Abstract

It is well recognized that vitamin D is necessary for optimal bone health. Emerging evidence is finding that vitamin D deficiency can have a profound effect on immunity, inflammation and muscle function. Studies in athletes have found that vitamin D status varies among different populations and is dependent on skin color, early- or late-day training, indoor training and geographic location. Although dietary assessment studies have found that athletes worldwide do not meet the dietary intake recommendations for vitamin D, the most probable reason for poor status is inadequate synthesis due to lack of sun exposure. Studies in athletic populations suggest that maintaining adequate vitamin D status may reduce stress fractures, total body inflammation, common infectious illnesses, and impaired muscle function, and may also aid in recovery from injury. Given that compromised vitamin D status can potentially impact an athlete's overall health and training efficiency, vitamin D status should be routinely assessed so that athletes can be coached to maintain serum 25(OH)D concentration of ≥30 and preferably ≥40 ng/ml. Recommendations will be dependent on the athlete's current 25(OH)D concentration, but can include regular safe sun exposure and/or dietary supplementation combined with increased vitamin D intake.

Copyright © 2013 Nestec Ltd., Vevey/S. Karger AG, Basel

Introduction

It has long been recognized that adequate vitamin D status is necessary for bone health and calcium regulation. Emerging evidence, however, indicates that vitamin D has other physiological roles which include immune and inflammatory modulation, and skeletal muscle function. In athletic populations, low vitamin D status has been linked to increased risk for stress fracture, acute respiratory infections and delayed recovery following surgery, all of which present a serious obstacle to training. This chapter discusses why and how coaching athletes to maintain adequate vitamin D status is a strategy to optimize health and ensure training efficiency.

Vitamin D Synthesis and Sources

Although vitamin D is labeled a 'vitamin', human needs can be met entirely through synthesis in the skin via exposure to sunlight [1, 2]. When ultraviolet radiation (UVB) hits the skin's surface, 7-dehydrocholesterol – present in the plasma membrane of skin cells – is converted to vitamin D_3 through a complex set of reactions. Newly synthesized vitamin D_3 is moved into circulation with the assistance of vitamin D-binding protein, and is subsequently converted to its main storage form, 25(OH)D, in the liver. Further conversion to the hormonally active form 1,25(OH)$_2$D in the kidney is driven by parathyroid hormone (PTH) when serum calcium and phosphate concentrations fall below physiological range. Many cells other than the kidney, also have the enzymatic machinery (1-α-hydroxylase) to produce 1,25(OH)$_2$D for use within that tissue (as explained below) [1]. Skin production of vitamin D, however, is variable and dependent on skin pigmentation, sunscreen use, skin area exposed, aging, cloud cover, wintertime latitude, and time of day of typical exposure. In winter months at latitudes greater than 35° North or South, vitamin D cannot be synthesized because the solar zenith angle prevents sufficient UVB from reaching the earth's surface.

Vitamin D is also obtained in the diet from limited natural and fortified sources including wild fatty fish, sun-dried mushrooms, egg yolks and fortified dairy, margarine and breakfast cereals (table 1). Dietary vitamin D includes both D_3 (cholecalciferol) and D_2 (ergocalciferol, derived from UVB exposure of fungi and yeast ergosterols). Both forms are readily absorbed (50% bioavailable) except in individuals with malabsorption disorders.

Vitamin D Status and Intake of Athletes

It is well recognized that vitamin D insufficiency and deficiency (see definitions, table 2) are widespread among the general population worldwide. Among athletes, the prevalence varies by sport, training location and skin color [3] and is higher in the winter and among athletes who train indoors. Athletes found to have the highest prevalence of vitamin D deficiency include gymnasts training

Table 1. Content of natural and fortified vitamin D-containing foods

Food	Serving size	Vitamin D, IU
Cod liver oil[1]	1 tsp	450
Wild salmon	3.5 oz	980
Swordfish	3.5 oz	670
Trout, steelhead	3.5 oz	604
Sun-dried mushroom powder (Dole)[2]	1 tsp	600
Mackerel, canned[1]	3.5 oz	290
Canned sardines[1]	3.5 oz	270
Farmed salmon	3.5 oz	249
Sun-dried mushrooms, raw[1]	½ cup	192
Tuna, light, canned[1]	3.5 oz	180
Yogurt, fortified[1]	1 cup	100–130
Milk, fortified[1]	8 oz	100
Orange juice, fortified[1]	8 oz	100
Tuna steak, yellow fin[1]	3.5 oz	82
Tuna, white, canned[1]	3.5 oz	80
Margarine, fortified[1]	1 tbsp	60
Cod, Atlantic[1]	3.5 oz	46
Cod, Pacific[1]	3.5 oz	24
Cereal, fortified (10% DV)[2]	¾ to 1 cup	40
Egg yolk[1]	1 whole	20–40

[1] Source: US Department of Agriculture, Agricultural Research Service. 2011. USDA National Nutrient Database for Standard Reference, release 24. Nutrient Data Laboratory home page, http://www.ars.usda.gov/nutrientdata.
[2] Selected food labels.

Table 2. Reference values for serum 25(OH)D

Category	Range, ng/ml
Deficient[1]	<20
Insufficient[2]	20–30 or 32
Sufficient[3]	>30 or 32
Optimal[4]	40–100
Toxic	>150 *plus* high serum calcium concentration

nmol/l = ng/ml × 2.5.
[1] Deficiency includes all concentrations below the approximate concentration where PTH begins to rise abruptly.
[2] Insufficiency includes all concentrations between deficiency and sufficiency.
[3] Sufficiency defined as the concentration where PTH plateaus and calcium absorption is maximized.
[4] Optimal is thought to be the serum 25(OH)D concentration where the human genome evolved and one where acute and chronic disease prevention is optimized.

in East Germany and Finland with 37–68% having serum 25(OH)D concentrations under 10–15 ng/ml, and Middle Eastern sportsmen training in Qatar of whom 91% were deficient [3]. On the other hand, only 12% of college athletes training in a mountainous region of the US had insufficient or deficient status in the fall [4].

Although the insufficient UVB exposure is the most probable explanation for suboptimal status, poor vitamin D intake may contribute. Studies over the last 15 years have found that an average vitamin D intake ranges from 100 IU to close to 250 IU/day [3, 4] in athletes across the globe. This falls short of the recommended intake of most counties. Higher vitamin D intake is expected in athletes who consume fatty fish several times per week, while lower intake is expected in those consuming few dairy products or fortified foods.

Functions of Vitamin D

As a secosteroid (i.e. steroids in which one of the steroid rings is opened), vitamin D functions as a modulator of several hundred genes [5–7]. In this process, cellular-derived 1,25(OH)$_2$D forms a complex with its nuclear vitamin D receptor and the retinoic acid x-receptor. This complex is recognized by specific elements on the gene sequence, and its binding acts as a switch to upregulate and downregulate (i.e. turn-on and turn-off) expression of specific genes [2]. This role as a genetic modulator switch explains why vitamin D plays a role in such a variety of physiologic functions – including bone health, muscle function, inflammation and immunity – all of which are important to training efficiency.

Bone Health
Vitamin D plays an important role in bone health by upregulating expression of genes that enhance intestinal calcium absorption and bone cell (osteoclast) activity [2]. In the general population, individuals who maintain higher D status have higher bone mineral density in the hip and lumbar spine and also optimize their ability to absorb dietary calcium and phosphorus. For example, 30–40% of dietary calcium and 80% of phosphorus is absorbed when serum 25(OH)D concentration is at least 30 ng/ml, but this drops to 10–15% of calcium and 60% of phosphorus in the vitamin D-insufficient state [2]. In active populations, sufficient vitamin D is important for stress fracture prevention. In Finnish military recruits, stress fracture risk was 3.6 times higher in those with insufficient status [25(OH)D concentration <30 ng/ml] compared to those with higher status [8]. A randomized double-blind, 8-week supplementation

trial found a 20% reduction in stress fracture incidence in female US naval recruits taking 800 IU plus 2,000 mg calcium compared to those taking a placebo [9].

Skeletal Muscle Function
Vitamin D is thought to influence muscle cell proliferation and differentiation, calcium and phosphate transport across the sarcolemma and muscle cell signaling through both gene expression modulation and nongenomic events. Animal studies have found that vitamin D deficiency induces atrophy of fast-twitch muscle fibers, impairs sarcoplasmic calcium uptake and prolongs time to peak contractile tension and relaxation [10]. Skeletal muscle pain and weakness – particularly in the proximal limbs – are well established but often forgotten symptoms of vitamin D deficiency that resolves with repletion [1, 2]. Recent studies in non-athletes living in the US, England and Saudi Arabia have found a link between vitamin D deficiency and persistent nonspecific musculoskeletal pain [11–13]. This pain has been shown to improve or resolve with vitamin D_3 supplementation that restores status [13].

Immunity and Inflammation
Vitamin D upregulates gene expression of specific broad-spectrum antimicrobial peptides (AMPs) – which are important regulators of immune defense – and also downregulates expression of inflammatory cytokines [1, 3]. Both are dependent on the circulating concentration of 25(OH)D, i.e. vitamin D status. AMPs, which include cathelecitin, are secreted by cells of the innate immune system including monocytes, macrophages, natural killer cells, and epithelial cells in the respiratory tract [14]. AMPs exert their effect by compromising the cell membrane integrity of invading bacteria, fungi and viruses. In clinical experiments, a single large dose of vitamin D_3 (100,000 IU) has been shown to enhance the innate immune response and restrict growth of the mycobacteria causing tuberculosis [15]. Vitamin D is also important in acquired immunity where it has an immunomodulatory effect on T and B lymphocytes.

An increasing number of studies in athletes and the general population have provided evidence that sufficient vitamin D status optimizes immune function and helps defend against acute respiratory illnesses including tuberculosis and the common cold. A large study in non-athletes found that maintaining a serum 25(OH)D of 38 ng/ml or higher reduced risk of developing an acute viral respiratory tract infection 2-fold, and reduced days missed from work [16]. A smaller study in college athletes found strikingly similar results. Athletes who maintained vitamin D status in the winter and spring that was at least 38 ng/ml had one or fewer episodes of illness, whereas those with lower stores had between one and four episodes. Finally, a randomized control trial involving postmenopausal nonathletic women showed that 1-year supplementation with 2,000 IU vitamin D nearly abolished the reported incidence of colds and flu [1].

Vitamin D also works through the immune system to control inflammation – which results from the accumulation of fluid and immune cells in injured tissue. Vitamin D increases production of several anti-inflammatory signaling molecules or cytokines including transforming growth factor and interleukin (IL)-4, and reduces production of several proinflammatory cytokines including IL-6 and tumor necrosis factor [3]. Several proinflammatory cytokines, particularly IL-6, are elevated following intense bouts of training, which unexplainably occurs to a greater degree in some well-trained athletes than others. Elevated concentrations of the proinflammatory cytokines are hypothesized to be involved in overtraining syndrome.

Currently, there is limited evidence that directly links compromised vitamin D status with increased risk or severity of sports-related inflammation, injury, or overtraining syndrome. The earliest recognition of this possibility, however, was mentioned in a 1950s German report which observed that athletes experienced a significant reduction in chronic pain due to sports injuries following 6 weeks of irradiation with a UVB-producing 'central sun lamp'. Another recently published study in distance runners found that vitamin D status was negatively associated with circulating concentrations of TNF-α (assessed 36 h after training), which was abruptly elevated as 25(OH)D concentration dropped below 32 ng/ml [3]. Another study in American professional football athletes found that players who sustained a muscle injury during the season had significant lower 25(OH)D concentration than those without muscle injury (19.9 vs. 24.7 ng/ml) [17].

Vitamin D Status and Athletic Performance

Given the role of vitamin D in skeletal muscle function, it is possible that vitamin D deficiency can compromise athletic performance. Published studies, however, have not evaluated whether vitamin D insufficiency or deficiency directly impairs muscle strength or performance in athletes. A recent review by Cannell et al. [5] presented provocative evidence from the Russian and German literature at the turn of the 20th century that UVB exposure improves athletic performance. These studies, however, did not measure vitamin D status and were not of rigorous scientific design compared to today's standards. Two recent studies in young nonathletic American women [18] and British school girls [19] with severely deficient status, however, observed positive associations between serum 25(OH)D concentration and both aerobic fitness [18], and jump height, velocity, and power [19]. A follow-up supplementation study in the British girls found that skeletal muscle movement efficiency, but not jumping performance, was improved after 1-year of supplementation which increased 25(OH)D concentration from 8 to 22 ng/ml [20]. Although it is not yet established whether there is a threshold above which skeletal muscle functions optimally, a study in active and sedentary older individuals observed steady increases in lower extremity muscle performance with increasing 25(OH)D concentration that plateaued around 38 ng/ml [21].

Vitamin D Status and Injury Rehabilitation

The importance of vitamin D status during musculoskeletal rehabilitation following injury or surgery is an emerging area of importance to athletes. Barker et al. [22] recently found that vitamin D status influenced strength and recovery in young, recreationally active individuals following anterior cruciate ligament repair. In this study, those with 25-OHD concentration below 30 ng/ml recovered more slowly and had significantly dampened increases in peak isometric force compared to those with concentrations above 30 ng/ml. Studies of patients in rehabilitation units are in support. One in a general rehabilitation unit found that vitamin D deficiency delayed rehabilitation and increased length of stay by 19% [23]. Another randomized trial in female stroke patients found that supplementation with 1,000 IU vitamin D/day improved muscle strength and increased the relative number and size of type II muscle fibers [24].

Vitamin D Requirements for Athletes

The recommended intake for vitamin D varies by country (table 3). The newly revised US and Canadian dietary recommendation is higher than those of most countries; however, many experts feel even these intake recommendations – which were established based exclusively on bone health [25] – are not high enough to promote optimal health [6] and may also not be high enough to optimize training efficiency. In fact, the Endocrine Society recommends that individuals with limited sun exposure require 1,500–2,000 IU/day to maintain sufficient status [6]. There is no evidence, however, that vitamin D needs are altered by physical training.

Table 3. Recommended vitamin D intake for children and adults

Group	Australia and New Zealand [27]	Nordic Countries [28]	UK [29]	US and Canada [25]	World Health Organization [30]
Children	200 (5)	300 (7.5)	280 (7), <4 years	600 (15)	200 (5)
Adolescents	200 (5)	300 (7.5)	from sun (400 if limited sun exposure)	600 (15)	200 (5)
Adults >18 or 19 years	200 (5)	300 (7.5)	from sun (400 if limited sun exposure)	600 (15)	200 (5)
Older adults	400 (10), 50–70 years 600 (15), >70 years	400 (10), >60 years	400	800 (20), >70 years	400 (10), 51–65 years 600 (15), >65 years

Recommendation provided as IU/day (μg/day is listed in parentheses).

Because dietary sources of vitamin D are limited, most athletes will need to meet requirements through regular supplementation, sensible sun exposure or a combination of dietary intake, sun exposure and supplementation. Regular consumption of vitamin D-fortified foods or a daily multivitamin alone is not likely to maintain sufficient status (>30 to 32 ng/ml) in the absence of regular UVB exposure.

Vitamin D Toxicity

Vitamin D toxicity is extremely rare [1]. It typically is observed with unintentional ingestion of extreme doses (i.e. well above 50,000 IU for longer than several months). Doses of 10,000 IU per day for up to 5 months, on the other hand, are shown to be safe [1]. Knowledge about vitamin D toxicity is important when working with athletes because some athletes, coaches and trainers believe that 'if a little is good, more is better'. Classic signs and symptoms of toxicity include fatigue, constipation, back pain, forgetfulness, nausea, vomiting, hypertension, heart rhythm abnormalities and tissue calcification (due to associated hypercalcemia). Vitamin D intoxication from UVB exposure, on the other hand, is not possible due to feedback loops which prevent synthesis of excess vitamin D_3 [25].

Vitamin D Assessment, Evaluation and Treatment

Routine screening for vitamin D deficiency should ensure that poor status does not compromise health and training efficiency. Bi- or tri-annual screening in association with training periodization, season and probable peak (late summer/early fall) and nadir (late winter) serum 25(OH)D concentrations may be most beneficial. If routine screening is not possible, athletes with a history of subpar performance, bone and joint injury (including stress fracture), skeletal weakness or pain, frequent illness or signs/symptoms of overtraining should be targeted.

Steps for assessing vitamin D status by the sports dietitian and members of the sports medicine team are outlined in table 4. Although serum 25(OH)D concentration (via a reliable assay) is the most important parameter, PTH and other biochemical indices may provide additional information when bone density is low or stress fracture (or reaction) is evident. PTH concentration increases in vitamin D deficiency and is independently related to bone density [4] and stress fracture risk [8] in athletic populations. The medical history and physical exam should address signs and symptoms of vitamin D deficiency. Documentation of current and recent medications is important because certain medications interfere with vitamin D absorption or metabolism [1, 2]. Dietary assessment should focus on estimating intake of vitamin D, as well as calcium and nutrients important to bone health and muscle function.

Following a detailed assessment, recommendations for achieving/maintaining optimal vitamin D status can be individualized to each athlete's 25(OH)D concentration, symptoms, diet, lifestyle habits and belief system. The recommendation to obtain 5 (in fair-skinned athletes) to 30 (in dark-skinned athletes) min of sunlight exposure to arms, legs and back several times a week at close to solar noon without sunscreen [1, 2] usually leads to sufficient vitamin D status. Fair-skinned individuals sunbathing in a bathing suit produce over 10,000 IU of vitamin D in less than 30 min [1]. Individuals with limited sun exposure require supplementation with at least 1,500–2,000 IU/day vitamin D to keep 25(OH)D concentrations in the sufficient range [6]. Higher doses may be required in those who have darker skin, and/or excess adiposity, malabsorption syndromes, or who take medications affecting vitamin D metabolism. Athletes who train at Northern/Sothern latitudes greater than 35° should supplement during winter even if they have adequate status during non-winter seasons. A recent study found that common genetic variants in vitamin D-binding protein predicted differences in response to D_3 supplementation [26], which help explain why some athletes do not respond to oral supplementation.

Table 4. Clinical assessment of vitamin D status

Anthropometrics and biological factors
- Age (synthesis efficiency decreased in those >60 years)
- Skin pigmentation (melanin absorbs UVB; dark-skinned individuals need longer exposure to make vitamin D)
- Body fat percentage (excess body fat is negatively correlated with vitamin D status)
- Weight history

Biochemical (laboratory) data
- Serum 25(OH)D concentration
- Other: PTH, alkaline phosphatase, serum calcium, serum phosphorus, serum magnesium, thyroid-stimulating hormone [useful if 25(OH)D is low]

Clinical
History
- Stress and other bone fracture(s)
- Bone pain
- Muscle pain, weakness, 'heaviness in legs'
- Chronic inflammatory or 'overuse' injuries
- Frequent acute illness or infection
- Overly sensitive to sun exposure
- Personal and/or family history of skin cancer/melanoma

Medications and supplements
- Anticonvulsants, corticosteroids, cimetidine, theophylline, orlistat, antituberculosis agents (may decrease vitamin D status)
- Thiazide diuretics, atorvastatin, other statins (may increase circulating vitamin D)
- Sulfonamides, phenothiazines, tetracyclines, psoralens, St. John's wort (increase sun sensitivity: may signal sun avoidance)
- Vitamin A supplementation (large quantities interfere with vitamin D metabolism)

Physical exam
- Unexplained musculoskeletal pain
- Muscle weakness (proximal limbs)
- Undue pain with pressure (thumb) on sternum or anterior tibia
- Knock knees, bowed legs, other lower limb deformities
- Bowel function (diarrhea, fat in stool)
- Skin pigmentation (or type)/hair color
- Contraindications to sunlight (albinism, porphyrias, xeroderma pigmentosum)

Dietary intake
- Vitamin D
- Vitamin D-containing supplements (including multivitamin)
- Calcium
- Phosphate (nutritional supplements and excess soda consumption may elevate PTH)
- Magnesium (commonly low in Western diet, important for muscle and bone health; deficiency may mask elevated PTH)
- Other nutrients: vitamins A, C and K, caffeine, omega-3/omega-6 fatty acids

Lifestyle and environmental
- Training regimen and environment in relation to sunlight exposure
- Training latitude, altitude, climate
- Sunscreen use (SPF of 15 ↓ synthesis capacity by >98%)
- Uniform or athletic clothing worn; SPF of clothing
- Leisure sun exposure (frequency, duration, and time of day)

Table 4. Continued

Lifestyle and environmental
- Tanning bed use (must emit UVB)
- Bathing habits after sun exposure (may rinse off skin cells containing newly synthesized vitamin D)
- Belief system (concerning sun exposure)

A modified version of this table was originally published in Larson-Meyer and Willis [3]. Permission was requested and granted.

To rapidly replenish stores, athletes with deficient status may benefit from short-term, high-dose 'loading' regimens under supervision of a physician. One such regimen involves treatment with 50,000 IU of vitamin D_2 or D_3 for at least 8 weeks to achieve a serum 25(OH)D concentration greater than 30 ng/ml followed by maintenance therapy of 1,500–2,000 IU/day [6]. High-dose treatment with cod liver oil is not recommended due to its high content of vitamin A. Although controversial, tanning beds which emit UVB can help maintain adequate vitamin D status [2, 4].

Conclusion

Recent research suggests that vitamin D plays a role in a vast array of physiological functions far beyond its well-known effects on bone metabolism, and these functions include immune and inflammatory modulation, and muscle function. Consequently, low vitamin D status could negatively impact the health and training efficiency of athletes. Research to date suggests that certain athletes are at risk for suboptimal vitamin D status, which may increase risk for stress fractures, acute illness, and suboptimal muscle function. Given these findings, it is important that sports dietitians routinely assess vitamin D status and make appropriate recommendations to coach athletes in achieving optimal status.

Disclosure Statement

The author declares that no financial or other conflict of interest exists in relation to the content of the chapter.

References

1 Cannell JJ, Hollis BW, Zasloff M, et al: Diagnosis and treatment of vitamin D deficiency. Expert Opin Pharmacother 2008;9:107–118.
2 Holick MF: Vitamin D deficiency. N Engl J Med 2007;357:266–281.
3 Willis KS, Smith DT, Broughton KS, Larson-Meyer DE: Vitamin D status and biomarkers of inflammation in runners. Open Access J Sports Med 2012;3:35042.
4 Halliday T, Peterson N, Thomas J, et al: Vitamin D status relative to diet, lifestyle, injury and illness in college athletes. Med Sci Sports Exerc 2011;42:335–343.
5 Cannell JJ, Hollis BW, Sorenson MB, et al: Athletic performance and vitamin D. Med Sci Sports Exerc 2009;41:1102–1110.
6 Holick MF, Binkley NC, Bischoff-Ferrari HA, et al: Evaluation, treatment, and prevention of vitamin D deficiency: an Endocrine Society clinical practice guideline. J Clin Endocrinol Metab 2011;96:1911–1930.
7 Zella LA, Shevde NK, Hollis BW, et al: Vitamin D-binding protein influences total circulating levels of 1,25-dihydroxyvitamin D3 but does not directly modulate the bioactive levels of the hormone in vivo. Endocrinology 2008;149:3656–3667.
8 Ruohola JP, Laaksi I, Ylikomi T, et al: Association between serum 25(OH)D concentrations and bone stress fractures in Finnish young men. J Bone Miner Res 2006;21:1483–1488.
9 Lappe J, Cullen D, Haynatzki G, et al: Calcium and vitamin D supplementation decreases incidence of stress fractures in female navy recruits. J Bone Miner Res 2008; 23:741–749.
10 Hamilton B: Vitamin D and human skeletal muscle. Scand J Med Sci Sports 2010;20:182–190.
11 Plotnikoff GA, Quigley JM: Prevalence of severe hypovitaminosis D in patients with persistent, nonspecific musculoskeletal pain. Mayo Clin Proc 2003;78:1463–1470.
12 Macfarlane GJ, Palmer B, Roy D, et al: An excess of widespread pain among South Asians: are low levels of vitamin D implicated? Ann Rheum Dis 2005;64:1217–1219.
13 Al Faraj S, Al Mutairi K: Vitamin D deficiency and chronic low back pain in Saudi Arabia. Spine 2003;28:177–179.
14 Gombart AF, Borregaard N, Koeffler HP: Human cathelicidin antimicrobial peptide (CAMP) gene is a direct target of the vitamin D receptor and is strongly up-regulated in myeloid cells by 1,25-dihydroxyvitamin D3. FASEB J 2005;19:1067–1077.
15 Martineau AR, Wilkinson RJ, Wilkinson KA, et al: A single dose of vitamin D enhances immunity to mycobacteria. Am J Respir Crit Care Med 2007;176:208–213.
16 Sabetta JR, DePetrillo P, Cipriani RJ, et al: Serum 25-hydroxyvitamin D and the incidence of acute viral respiratory tract infections in healthy adults. PLoS One 2010; 5:e11088.
17 Shindle M, Voos J, Gulotta L, et al: Vitamin D status in a professional American football team. Med Sci Sports Exerc 2011;43:S340–S341.
18 Mowry DA, Costello MM, Heelan KA: Association among cardiorespiratory fitness, body fat, and bone marker measurements in healthy young females. J Am Osteopath Assoc 2009;109:534–539.
19 Ward KA, Das G, Berry JL, et al: Vitamin D status and muscle function in post-menarchal adolescent girls. J Clin Endocrinol Metab 2009;94:559–563.
20 Ward KA, Das G, Roberts SA, et al: A randomized, controlled trial of vitamin D supplementation upon musculoskeletal health in postmenarchal females. J Clin Endocrinol Metab 2010;95:4643–4651.
21 Bischoff-Ferrari HA, Dietrich T, Orav EJ, et al: Higher 25-hydroxyvitamin D concentrations are associated with better lower-extremity function in both active and inactive persons aged > or = 60 y. Am J Clin Nutr 2004;80:752–758.
22 Barker T, Martins TB, Hill HR, et al: Low vitamin D impairs strength recovery after anterior cruciate ligament surgery. J Evid Based Complementary Altern Med 2011;16: 201–209.
23 Kiebzak GM, Moore NL, Margolis S, et al: Vitamin D status of patients admitted to a hospital rehabilitation unit: relationship to function and progress. Am J Phys Med Rehabil 2007;86:435–445.

24 Sato Y, Iwamoto J, Kanoko T, et al: Low-dose vitamin D prevents muscular atrophy and reduces falls and hip fractures in women after stroke: a randomized controlled trial. Cerebrovasc Dis 2005;20:187–192.

25 Ross AC, Taylor CL, Yaktine AL, et al: Dietary Reference Intakes for Calcium and Vitamin D. Washington, National Academies Press, 2010, p 482.

26 Fu L, Yun F, Oczak M, et al: Common genetic variants of the vitamin D binding protein (DBP) predict differences in response of serum 25-hydroxyvitamin D [25(OH)D] to vitamin D supplementation. Clin Biochem 2009;42:1174–1177.

27 The Australian National Health and Medical Research Council (NHMRC) and the New Zealand Ministry of Health: Nutrient Reference Values for Australia and New Zealand Commonwealth of Australia, 2006.

28 Nordic Nutrition Recommendations 2004: Integrating Nutrition and Physical Activity, ed 4. Copenhagen, Nordic Council of Ministers, 2004.

29 Department of Health. Committee on the Medical Aspects of Food Policy (COMA): Report on Dietary Reference Values for Food Energy and Nutrients for the United Kingdom. London, HMSO, 1991.

30 World Health Organization, Food and Agricultural Organization of the United Nations: Vitamin and Mineral Requirements in Human Nutrition. Geneva, WHO Publications, 2004.

Weight Management in the Performance Athlete

Melinda M. Manore

School of Biological and Population Sciences, Nutrition and Exercise, College of Public Health and Human Sciences, Oregon State University, Corvallis, OR, USA

Abstract

Management of weight is an ever-increasing challenge in societies where good tasting food is convenient, relatively inexpensive, and abundant. Developing a weight management plan is essential for everyone, including athletes that expend high amounts of energy in their sport. This brief review addresses the concept of dynamic energy balance and dietary approaches that can be successfully used with active individuals to facilitate weight loss, while retaining lean tissue and minimizing risks for disordered eating. Emphasis is placed on teaching athletes the benefits of consuming a low-energy-dense diet (e.g. high-fiber, high-water, low-fat foods), which allows for the consumption of a greater volume of food that is satiating but reduces energy intake. Other dietary behaviors important for weight loss or weight maintenance after weight loss are also emphasized, such as eating breakfast, spreading food and protein intake throughout the day, eating after exercise, elimination of sweetened beverages, and avoiding fad diets. As the general population becomes heavier, more young athletes will come to their sport needing to alter bodyweight or composition to perform at their peak. Health professionals need to be prepared with effective and evidence-based dietary approaches to help the athletes achieve their bodyweight goals.

Copyright © 2013 Nestec Ltd., Vevey/S. Karger AG, Basel

Introduction

Achieving energy balance and maintaining bodyweight should be easy – balance energy intake with energy expenditure. Achieving weight loss also appears to be simple – just increase energy expenditure and/or reduce energy intake. So why isn't it simple? Why don't people lose or gain lean tissue as we predict from our calculations? Many athletes have weight concerns, they frequently want to lose weight to be competitive and improve performance, while maintaining or gaining lean tissue. They also differ from the sedentary overweight individuals because they are already active, and increasing exercise or altering their training routine may not be an option. This brief review will primarily address dietary approaches that can be successfully used with active individuals to facilitate weight loss, while retaining lean tissue. Of course, any approach to weight loss also needs to minimize the risk of disordered eating behaviors and pathogenic weight loss practices that can arise when an athlete is dieting. This review will not address weight gain in athletes, which has been reviewed elsewhere [1].

Achieving a Healthy Bodyweight

The need or desire to lose weight and/or change body composition is common among competitive and recreational athletes. As the number of young overweight and obese individuals increase in the population, more young athletes will come to their sport heavier, which may increase the pressure placed on them to lose weight to be competitive. This also means the amount of weight loss needed to reach a competitive and/or healthy weight and body composition may be higher. Although the overweight or obese athlete may not approach weight loss for the health benefits, for these athletes weight loss can reduce the risk of chronic disease, and improve their overall health and ability to participate in sport. For example, Borchers et al. [2] found that 21% of their division 1 college football players (mean age = 20 years) were obese (≥25% body fat) and had insulin resistance, while 9% had metabolic syndrome (all obese). Currently, approximately 66% of the US adult population is either overweight and/or obese, with ~34% being obese [3, 4]. The overweight and obesity rates in US children are also high, which means more children and young adults participating in sports will be heavier [5]. Unfortunately, obesity is a worldwide problem, and the high rates of obesity seen in the US are mimicked in other developed countries around the world [6].

Conversely, there are those elite and recreational athletes, who based on either body mass index (BMI) or body composition data, are at normal weight or have low bodyweights. Yet, these individuals also want to lose weight for their sport to improve performance and/or to achieve an aesthetically pleasing body shape. Some of these individuals are young and still growing, which is the least desirable time to severely restrict energy intake, while participating in high lev-

Table 1. Thermogenesis induced by nutrients in humans and the cost of nutrient storage

Nutrient	Thermogenesis, %	Cost of nutrient storage, %
Glucose	6–8	12
Lipid	3	4
Amino acids	25–40	25–40

Adapted from Manore et al. [12].

els of exercise. At the same time, it is imperative that the risk of introducing disordered eating behaviors is minimized, especially in those athletes participating in lean build sports [7]. Finally, it can be difficult to manage safe weight loss in athletes who need to meet a designated weight on competition day, such as lightweight rowers, jockeys or wrestlers. Few athletes are naturally lightweight enough for these types of competitive sports, so weight loss will be required the weeks or days prior to competition [8].

What is the best approach to manage weight and weight loss in these different groups – those who are already lean and want to be leaner, while retaining lean tissue, and those who are overweight, who need to lose body fat but also want to retain lean tissue?

Energy Balance – Understanding the Factors

The classic energy balance equation states that if energy intake (total kcals consumed) equals energy expenditure (total kcals expended), then weight is maintained. Although the concept of energy balance appears simple, it is a dynamic process [9]. Changing one factor on the energy intake side can also impact factors on the energy expenditure side. Thus, numerous factors are working together to influence each side of the energy balance equation, which ultimately determines bodyweight. For example, total energy expenditure will be influenced by total energy intake and macronutrient composition of the diet, which can change the thermic effect of food (see table 1) and substrate oxidation during exercise [10–12]. Conversely, high-intensity exercise can blunt appetite-regulating hormones, which could reduce energy intake [13, 14]. Another factor that can confound the assessment of energy needs is the total amount of non-sport-related activities (e.g. walking, biking for transpiration, etc.) and the amount sitting, standing and fidgeting an athlete does [15]. While some athletes are very active outside of training for their sport, others become quite sedentary when they are not training, which can decrease energy needs below predicted levels [16].

A common mistake made by many health professionals when explaining energy balance to athletes is to assume that changing either side of the equation by 3,500 kcal (7,700 kJ) will always result in a pound (~0.5 kg) of weight gained or lost, without considering all the other factors that might change as energy intake or energy expenditure is altered. A classic example of this concept was illustrated by Swinburn and Ravussin [17]. They demonstrated what would happen to a 75-kg man who consumed an extra 100 kcal/day (~420 kJ) every day for 40 years. Using the static energy balance equation this amount of extra energy would equal ~1.5 million kcals or an estimated weight gain of 417 pounds (~190 kg) over this period. Yet this does not happen. This simple calculation does not take into account the increase in energy expenditure that would occur, including increased resting metabolic rate, as weight increased. Thus, after a short period of positive energy balance, bodyweight would increase, resulting in an increase in energy expenditure that will eventually balance the increased energy intake. The individual would then achieve energy balance and become weight stable at a higher bodyweight. Thus, the extra 100 kcal/day would result in a more realistic weight gain of ~6 pounds (~2.7 kg). To maintain this larger body size, the individual would need to continue to eat these additional kcals. Of course, the amount of weight gained will depend on the number of extra kcals consumed, the composition of these kcals (i.e. the amount of fat, carbohydrate, protein, or alcohol), and overall energy expenditure.

Figure 1 illustrates this complex concept by showing some of the factors that can influence each side of the energy balance equation, which ultimately determine bodyweight. Some of these factors include genetics, changes in regulatory hormones that control energy balance and appetite, gut health, and the food and exercise environment that can drive eating, exercise and body composition. For a more detailed explanation of these factors, see Galgani and Ravussin [9].

Achieving a Healthy Bodyweight

Determining an optimal or healthy weight for an athlete competing in a sport is difficult because no charts or tables provide the answer. However, the following criteria are frequently used to help determine a person's healthy bodyweight, regardless of his/her activity level [12]. This list might help the athlete determine what weight works best for him/her during the off-season and amount of time

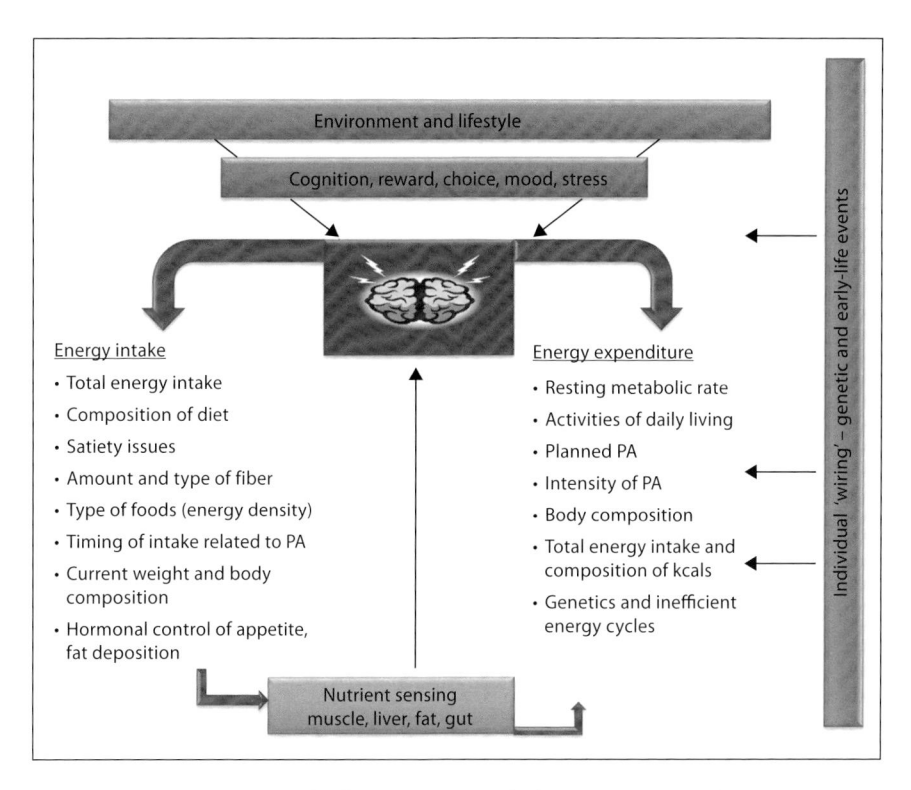

Fig. 1. Factors regulating and influencing energy balance. PA = Physical activity.

and energy required to maintain a lower bodyweight during the competitive season, while remaining healthy and injury free.
- Weight that minimizes health risks and promotes good health and eating habits, while allowing for optimal training and performance in one's sport.
- Weight that takes into consideration genetic makeup and family history of body weight and shape.
- Weight that is appropriate for age and level of physical development, including normal reproductive function in women.
- Weight that can be accepted by the individual and be maintained without constant dieting or restraining food intake, which could lead to disordered eating or an eating disorder.

Thus, optimal bodyweight should promote good health and be 'reasonable' in terms of whether or not it can be achieved and maintained. If an individual is constantly dieting or repeatedly gaining and losing weight, they may be trying to achieve or maintain an unrealistic bodyweight. Conversely, in sports that require a low bodyweight, an athlete may purposefully drop to a lighter weight during periods of high competition or choose to compete at a lower weight class. For example, a ski jumper, wrestler or cyclists will be lighter during the competitive season, while gaining weight during the off-season, since it is unrealistic, and unhealthy, to maintain a low bodyweight the entire year. While it is important for athletes to achieve and maintain a healthy bodyweight throughout the year, some athletes will target bodyweights that are difficult to maintain after competition. Thus, it is important for these athletes to regain some weight during the off-season, but not so much that severe weight loss is required for the next competitive season. It is also important to prevent disordered eating in athletes, which requires that the athlete maintain healthy eating habits. It also requires that the medical and coaching staff know and can recognize risk factors for disordered eating when they occur and initiate early intervention if necessary [7].

Targeting Weight Loss: Dietary Strategies for Athletes

What dietary and physical activity behaviors/changes will produce the desired body composition and weight changes, while being sustainable and manageable by the individual? Although the answers will be different depending on the individual and his/her sport, the following section highlights diet behaviors with research to support their recommendation to athletes who are interested in losing weight, maintaining lean tissue and prevention of weight regain. This section does not address changes in exercise strategies or training routines since the coach typically determines these for the athlete. Since athletes are already active, they will need to rely more heavily on the dietary strategies listed below to achieve weight loss.

Adopt a Low-Energy-Dense Diet Plan
A low-energy-dense diet is a diet that is high in whole fruits and vegetables, whole grains, and incorporates low-fat dairy, legumes/beans, and lean meats. Overall, the diet is low in fat and reduces or eliminates beverages containing calories, especially sweetened beverages and alcohol. This high-fiber, high-water, low-fat diet means an individual can consume a greater volume of food for an overall lower energy intake and still feel satiated. The energy density of a diet or a food is determined by measuring the amount of energy (kcals) for a given amount (g) of food (kcal/day). Evidence shows that a low-energy-density eating plan is effective at reducing energy intake, facilitating weight loss and prevention of weight regain, and maintaining satiety in well-controlled feeding studies and in free-living conditions [18, 19]. For example, Bell et al. [20] examined the effectiveness of a low-energy-density eating plan on energy intake and weight

loss. They found that when they fed three different levels of energy-dense diets, the women ate a similar amount and weight of food, but on the lowest low-energy dense diet condition, participants consumed 30% less energy than the high-energy density diet. Furthermore, the women did not report any differences in hunger and fullness ratings or enjoyment of the meals across test conditions. In a follow-up study, Rolls et al. [21] examined the effect of changing portion size, energy density or a combination of the two conditions on total energy intake over a 2-day period. Energy density was altered by changing the portions of vegetables in entrées and by substituting low-fat foods/ingredients for full-fat foods (e.g. skim milk for whole milk). They found that energy density and portion size independently altered energy intake. When portion size was reduced by 25%, energy intake decreased by 231 kcal/day (10% decrease); however, reducing energy density by 25% decreased energy intake by 575 kcal/day (24% decrease). When both energy density and portion sizes were reduced simultaneously, energy intake decreased by 32%. Thus, reducing portion sizes and energy density dramatically reduce energy intake; however, just reducing the energy density of the foods consumed reduces energy intake more than reducing portion sizes.

Overall, reducing the energy density of the diet is more effective at lowering energy intake than reducing portion size, without effecting hunger, fullness, or enjoyment of the food. For athletes trying to lose weight, this has important implications. It may be easier for an active individual to consume a similar amount of food and focus on changing the energy density rather than portion sizes. This approach reduces hunger and increases adherence to the weight loss diet plan. Finally, following a lower energy-dense diet can help the athlete maintain his/her weight loss.

In summary, a key component of a low-energy-density eating plan is to increase intake of foods high in water and fiber to promote satiation, while reducing both high-fat foods (i.e. potato chips, cheese, cookies) and low water and fiber foods (i.e. baked tortilla chips, pretzels). Consumption of low-fat, low-water, low-fiber foods are not as satiating. Another advantage of the low-energy-density plan is that it increased total fiber intake, which also increases sense of fullness and helps individuals achieve adequate dietary fiber.

Eating Breakfast and Timing of Meals
For the athlete, timing of food intake around exercise training and spreading food intake throughout the day will assure that the body has the energy and nutrients needed for exercise and the building and repair of lean tissue. This approach can also prevent the athlete from becoming too hungry and consuming foods or beverages not on their diet plan.

A growing body of research evidence shows that eating breakfast is associated with a lower energy intake and bodyweight and better diet quality and weight management [22, 23]. For example, Astbury et al. [24] found that men who ate breakfast consumed 17% fewer kcals at lunch. Data from the National Weight Control Registry also show that 80% of individuals who had lost at least 30 pounds (6.6 kg) and kept the weight of for at least one year were breakfast eaters [25]. Skipping breakfast may lead to an upregulation of appetite, which could lead to weight gain over time [23]. For the athlete, breakfast is especially important; it helps replenish glycogen after an overnight fast and provides fuel for exercise. Fortunately, it is easy to consume a low-energy-dense, high-nutrient-dense breakfast by including low-fat high-quality protein (e.g. low-fat dairy or soy products, egg whites, lean meats) and fiber- and nutrient-rich foods (e.g. whole grains and fruits).

Athletes also need to consume adequate high-quality protein throughout the day, but especially after exercise and at breakfast [26]. This dietary approach can benefit the athlete trying to lose weight in two ways. First, it assures that adequate protein is available for building, repair and maintenance of lean tissue throughout the day. Second, higher protein diets have been associated with increased satiety and reductions in energy intake. For example, Weigle et al. [27] reported a decrease in energy intake (–441 ± 64 kcal/day) over a 12-week period in individuals (BMI = 26.2 ± 2.1) fed an ad libitum high-protein diet (30% energy from protein; 20% fat and 50% carbohydrate) compared to an isocaloric lower protein diet (15% of energy from protein). Although most athletes get plenty of protein [12], they may not be strategic about getting this protein after exercise and spreading it out across the day. It may be more typical for the majority of the energy and protein to come in a large meal at the end of the day. Finally, it is important that protein intake remain high, even when energy is being restricted for weight loss. For active individuals not attempting weight loss, the recommended protein intake is 1.2–1.7 g protein/kg [28]. When energy is restricted, protein intake may need to be higher than this to help maintain lean tissue and preserve strength. For example, Mettler et al. [29] fed 60% of habitual energy intake to lean (16% body fat) resistance-trained males for 2 weeks. One group consumed 15% of energy from protein (~1 g/kg), while another group received 35% of energy from protein (~2.3 g/kg). At the end of the 2 week period, the 35% energy from protein group maintained their lean mass (–0.3 kg), with the majority of weight loss coming from fat while the 15% energy from protein group lost significantly more lean body mass (–1.6 kg). These data strongly suggest that when lean fit individuals reduce energy intake for weight loss while continuing to maintain a high level of physical activity, protein intake may need to be higher that typically recommended.

Refueling after exercise is still important for the athlete who wants to lose weight. Thus, the post-exercise dietary routine needs to include fluids for rehydration, carbohydrate in the form of low-energy-dense foods (e.g. whole fruits and vegetables, whole grains) to replenish glycogen, and high-quality low-fat protein for building and repair of lean tissue. Because many athletes may not have these foods readily available after exercise, they must plan ahead and strategically use sport foods and/or health snacks to meet their energy and nutrient needs while staying within their diet plan. A sport dietitian can teach the athlete how to shop, select and prepare low-energy-dense foods.

Reduce Intake of High-Calorie Beverages

High-calorie sweetened beverages and alcohol can derail any athlete trying to lose weight. They add extra energy to the diet without increasing satiety or reducing the amount of food consumed with these beverages [30]. For some athletes, just the elimination of high-calorie beverages from their diet (e.g. soda, alcohol, fruit juice, energy drinks, or flavored coffee/teas) could help them achieve their weight loss goals without making any other dietary changes.

Avoid Fad Diets

Although it is tempting for both the athlete and coach to use extreme diet practices that result in rapid weight loss, these diets should be avoided. Combining severe energy restriction with an intense endurance and strength training program can actually result in metabolic adaptations that diminish the additive effects of these two factors on weight loss [31] while being extremely stressful for the athlete. In addition, Garthe et al. [32] also showed that slower more reasonable weight loss in athletes (~0.7% loss of bodyweight/week) helped preserve lean tissue while improving strength gains over more severe weight loss (1.4% weight loss/week). Finally, severe energy restriction has a number of other negative consequences for the athletes that are bulleted below [12]:

- Decreased ability to train at higher intensities due to poor energy intake and glycogen replacement resulting in decreased aerobic and anaerobic performance.
- Increased risk of injury due to fatigue and loss of lean tissue.
- Increased risk of disordered eating behaviors due to severe energy restriction.
- Increased risk of dehydration, especially if the diet is ketogenic.
- Increased risk of poor nutrient intakes, including essential nutrients, due to limited food intake.
- Increased emotional distress due to hunger, fatigue and stress of following an energy-restricted diet.

Conclusions

Management of weight is an ever-increasing challenge in societies where good tasting food is convenient, relatively inexpensive, and abundant. Developing a weight management plan is essential for everyone, including athletes that expend high amounts of energy in their sport. Weight loss can be difficult and may change body composition unfavorably; thus, managing weight during the off-season is especially important to avoid performance-damaging rapid weight loss during competition. Weight management plans need to be individualized considering both the sport and the weight loss goals. This may require a multidisciplinary approach that includes the athlete, coach, sports medicine team and sport dietitian. Finally, it is imperative that health professionals understand the many physiological and environmental factors influencing bodyweight. This will improve their ability to design individualized and realistic weight management programs.

Disclosure Statement

The author declares that no financial or other conflict of interest exists in relation to the content of the chapter.

References

1 Rankin JW: Weight loss and gain in athletes. Curr Sports Med Rep 2002;1:208–213.
2 Borchers JR, Clem KL, Habash DL, et al: Metabolic syndrome and insulin resistance in Division 1 collegiate football players. Med Sci Sports Exerc 2009;41:2105–2110.
3 Flegal KM, Carroll MD, Ogden CL, Curtin LR: Prevalence and trends in obesity among US adults, 1999–2008. JAMA 2010;303:235–241.
4 Ogden CL, Carroll MD: Prevalence of overweight, obesity and extreme obesity among adults: United States, Trends 1960–1962 through 2007–2008. National Center for Health Statistics 2010. http://www.cdc.gov/nchs/fastats/overwt.htm.
5 Ogden CL, Carroll MD, Curtin LR, et al: Prevalence of high body mass index in US children and adolescents, 2007–2008. JAMA 2010;303:242–249.
6 Swinburn BA, Sacks G, Hall KD, et al: The global obesity pandemic: shaped by global drivers and local environments. Lancet 2011; 378:804–814.
7 Sundgot-Borgen J, Torstveit MK: Aspects of disordered eating continuum in elite high-intensity sports. Scand J Med Sci Sports 2010;2:112–121.
8 Slater GJ, Rice AJ, Sharpe K, et al: Body-mass management of Australian lightweight rowers prior to and during competition. Med Sci Sports Exerc 2005;37:860–866.
9 Galgani J, Ravussin E: Energy metabolism, fuel selection and body weight regulation. Int J Obesity 2008;32(suppl 7):S109–S119.
10 Hawley JA, Burke LM, Phillips SM, Spriet LL: Nutritional modulation of training-induced skeletal muscle adaptations. J Appl Physiol 2011;110:834–845.

11 Hawley JA, Burke LM: Carbohydrate availability and training adaptation: effects on cell metabolism. Exerc Sport Sci Rev 2010;38:152–160.
12 Manore MM, Meyer NL, Thompson J: Sport Nutrition for Health and Performance, ed 2. Champaign, Human Kinetics, 2009.
13 Stensel D: Exercise, appetite and appetite-regulating hormones: implications for food intake and weight control. Ann Nutr Metab 2010;2:36–42.
14 Hagobian TA, Braun B: Physical activity and hormonal regulation of appetite: sex differences and weight control. Exerc Sport Sci Rev 2010;38:25.
15 Levine JA: Non-exercise activity thermogenesis (NEAT). Nutr Rev 2004;62:S82–S97.
16 Thompson J, Manore M, Skinner J: Resting metabolic rate and thermic effect of a meal in low-and adequate-energy intake male endurance athletes. Int J Sport Nutr 1993;3:194.
17 Swinburn B, Ravussin E: Energy balance or fat balance? Am J Clin Nutr 1993;57:770S–771S.
18 Rolls BJ: The relationship between dietary energy density and energy intake. Physiol Behav 2009;97:609–615.
19 Ello-Martin JA, Ledikwe JH, Rolls BJ: The influence of food portion size and energy density on energy intake: implications for weight management. Am J Clin Nutr 2005;82:236S–241S.
20 Bell EA, Castellanos VH, Pelkman CL, et al: Energy density of foods affects energy intake in normal-weight women. Am J Clin Nutr 1998;67:412.
21 Rolls BJ, Roe LS, Meengs JS: Reductions in portion size and energy density of foods are additive and lead to sustained decreases in energy intake. Am J Clin Nutr 2006;83:11–17.
22 Timlin MT, Pereira MA: Breakfast frequency and quality in the etiology of adult obesity and chronic diseases. Nutr Rev 2007;65:268–281.
23 Pereira MA, Erickson E, McKee P, et al: Breakfast frequency and quality may affect glycemia and appetite in adults and children. J Nutr 2011;141:163–168.
24 Astbury NM, Taylor MA, Macdonald IA: Breakfast consumption affects appetite, energy intake, and the metabolic and endocrine responses to foods consumed later in the day in male habitual breakfast eaters. J Nutr 2011;141:1381–1389.
25 Wyatt HR, Grunwald GK, Mosca CL, et al: Long-term weight loss and breakfast in subjects in the National Weight Control Registry. Obes Res 2002;10:78–82.
26 Westerterp-Plantenga MS, Nieuwenhuizen A, Tomé D, et al: Dietary protein, weight loss, and weight maintenance. Annu Rev Nutr 2009;29:21–41.
27 Weigle DS, Breen PA, Matthys CC, et al: A high-protein diet induces sustained reductions in appetite, ad libitum caloric intake, and body weight despite compensatory changes in diurnal plasma leptin and ghrelin concentrations. Am J Clin Nutr 2005;82:41.
28 Rodriguez NR, DiMarco NM, Langley S: Nutrition and athletic performance. Med Sci Sports Exerc 2009;41:709–731.
29 Mettler S, Mitchell N, Tipton KD: Increased protein intake reduces lean body mass loss during weight loss in athletes. Med Sci Sports Exerc 2010;42:326–337.
30 Malik VS, Schulze MB, Hu FB: Intake of sugar-sweetened beverages and weight gain: a systematic review. Am J Clin Nutr 2006;84:274–288.
31 Donnelly JE, Blair SN, Jakicic JM, et al, American College of Sports Medicine: American College of Sports Medicine Position Stand. Appropriate physical activity intervention strategies for weight loss and prevention of weight regain for adults. Med Sci Sports Exerc 2009;41:459–471.
32 Garthe I, Raastad T, Refsnes PE, et al: Effect of two different weight-loss rates on body composition and strength and power-related performance in elite athletes. Int J Sport Nutr Exerc Metab 2011;21:97–104.

Tipton KD, van Loon LJC (eds): Nutritional Coaching Strategy to Modulate Training Efficiency.
Nestlé Nutr Inst Workshop Ser, vol 75, pp 135–141, (DOI: 10.1159/000345862)
Nestec Ltd., Vevey/S. Karger AG., Basel, © 2013

Concluding Remarks: Nutritional Strategies to Support the Adaptive Response to Prolonged Exercise Training

Luc J.C. van Loon[a] · Kevin D. Tipton[b]

[a]Department of Human Movement Sciences, NUTRIM School for Nutrition, Toxicology and Metabolism, Maastricht University Medical Centre+, Maastricht, The Netherlands;
[b]Health and Exercise Sciences Research Group, University of Stirling, Stirling, UK

Abstract

Nutrition plays a key role in allowing the numerous training hours to be translated into useful adaptive responses of various tissues in the individual athlete. Research over the last decade has shown many examples of the impact of dietary interventions to modulate the skeletal muscle adaptive response to prolonged exercise training. Proper nutritional coaching should be applied throughout both training and competition, each with their specific requirements regarding nutrient provision. Such dietary support will improve exercise training efficiency and, as such, further increase performance capacity. Here, we provide an overview on the properties of various nutritional interventions that may be useful to support the adaptive response to exercise training and competition and, as such, to augment exercise training efficiency.

Copyright © 2013 Nestec Ltd., Vevey/S. Karger AG, Basel

Introduction

In addition to regular exercise training, diet represents a key factor that modulates exercise performance. A healthy diet, designed to meet the specific demands imposed upon by the individual athlete's training and competition, is required to allow maximal performance. Most athletes are preoccupied with diet and nutritional support to meet nutrient requirements prior to and during exercise competition. As a result, nutritional interventions, with or without the use of specifically designed sports nutrition products, are now generally applied to compensate for the metabolic demands imposed upon by intense exercise competition. However, there is an increasing awareness that diet also plays a key role in translating the many training hours into useful adaptive responses of various tissues in the individual athlete. Research over the last decade has uncovered many examples of the impact of various dietary interventions to modulate the skeletal muscle adaptive response to prolonged exercise training. Of course, this modulation by nutrition is not unexpected as the adaptive response to each successive exercise bout ultimately determines the training status of the athlete, thereby allowing peak performance. Consequently, proper nutritional coaching is not something that should be restricted to the competitive events, as it needs to be applied throughout both training as well as competition. Proper nutritional support will likely optimize the ability to train effectively and ultimately increase performance capacity. The aim of this workshop was to explore the numerous properties of various nutritional interventions that may help to support the adaptive response to exercise training and, as such, to identify nutritional strategies that may improve exercise training efficiency.

Nutritional Strategies to Modulate Exercise Training Efficiency

Manipulating Carbohydrate Availability
Endogenous glycogen stores are, from a quantitative point of view, the most important substrate source during moderate- to high-intensity endurance type exercise. To optimize performance during competition, athletes generally aim to maximize endogenous and exogenous carbohydrate availability. However, in their build-up to competition, most competitive athletes follow an intricate periodization of diet and training load. In this process, athletes tend to experiment with the systematic manipulation of endogenous carbohydrate availability. Nutrient availability has been well recognized as a key factor regulating the adaptive response to exercise training. In the chapter 'Nutritional Strategies to Modulate the Adaptive Response to Endurance Training', *John Hawley* discusses the application of training sessions in which carbohydrate availability is intentionally reduced, often referred to as 'training low'. Exercise sessions performed under these conditions generally show a (more) massive upregulation of various markers of training adaptation. However, under such low glycogen availability, the total workload or workload intensity of a training session can be severely compromised. Therefore, training under low glycogen availability is unlikely of benefit when performed exclusively. However, decreasing glycogen availability through dietary interventions before, during, and/or after a subset of exercise

training sessions may represent an effective strategy to further enhance the adaptive response to endurance type exercise training. It will be of interest to define the optimal nutrient-training regimen that can enhance endurance training efficiency and improve subsequent performance.

Bicarbonate Loading
For many decades, athletes have been experimenting with sodium bicarbonate to increase the capacity for extracellular buffering of hydrogen ions to improve performance capacity during relatively short bouts of exhaustive exercise. In the chapter 'Practical Considerations for Bicarbonate Loading and Sports Performance', an overview is provided on the practical issues when aiming to improve performance capacity by using sodium bicarbonate. Consuming a small (300 mg/kg) amount of sodium bicarbonate prior to exercise can effectively improve performance capacity in sports activities during which intense exercise is sustained for 1–7 min. Despite the convincing ergogenic properties of sodium bicarbonate use to improve subsequent performance capacity, there is very little research that investigates the impact of more prolonged sodium bicarbonate (or any other hydrogen buffer) use on the adaptive response to more prolonged exercise training. A greater training intensity, facilitated by the greater hydrogen ion buffer capacity, might further enhance the adaptive response to prolonged interval training efficiency. The latter could be of considerable relevance to those athletes that require a rapid and sustained increase in performance capacity during more intense, intermittent type exercise activities.

Dietary Nitrate
A similar rationale can be used for the ergogenic properties of dietary nitrate. Over the last decade, we have been confronted with the interesting ergogenic properties of dietary nitrate. In the chapter 'Influence of Dietary Nitrate Supplementation on Exercise Tolerance and Performance', *Andrew Jones* presents an overview on the proposed impact of supplementing inorganic nitrate on pulmonary oxygen uptake. A reduced oxygen cost of exercise activities such as cycling, walking, running and knee extension exercise have been reported following nitrate supplementation. The latter also seems to translate to an increase in exercise performance, as greater time to exhaustion and increased time trial performance have recently been reported following a few days of nitrate supplementation. Though there is a renewed interest in the potential ergogenic properties of nitrate, there is still much to be learned. Besides establishing the physiological mechanism(s) responsible for the ergogenic properties of dietary nitrate supplementation, we need to establish the various modalities that define the proposed ergogenic properties of dietary nitrate in various different exercise

activities. Subsequently, it is of interest to speculate on the impact of more prolonged nitrate supplementation as a means to modulate exercise training efficiency.

High-Intensity Exercise Training

High-intensity exercise training (HIT) has been identified as an efficient exercise modality to allow rapid skeletal muscle adaptation to augment oxidative and non-oxidative metabolism with a minimal amount of time spent exercising. In his chapter 'Nutritional Strategies to Support Adaptation to High Intensity Interval Training in Team Sports', *Martin Gibala* speculates on the capacity of nutritional interventions to further enhance the benefits of intermittent HIT. So far, the focus of the research on HIT has been on establishing the physiological mechanisms responsible for the rapid skeletal muscle adaptive response. Future work is warranted to assess whether ergogenic aids, such as sodium bicarbonate, β-alanine and/or inorganic nitrate, may be applied effectively to augment HIT-induced physiological remodeling and/or promote greater performance adaptations.

Recovery from Injury

Injury is generally an unavoidable aspect of sports participation. As a consequence, injury and subsequent recovery represents an integrative role in exercise training and the preparation for competition. Limb immobilization following injury has profound implications for muscle and tendon metabolism, leading to the loss of muscle mass, strength, and function. In the chapter 'Dietary Strategies to Attenuate Muscle Loss during Recovery from Injury' various nutritional strategies are proposed by *Kevin Tipton* that may attenuate the loss of muscle tissue during a period of immobilization or reduced physical activity due to injury or disease. Maintenance of a healthy diet, including the consumption of ample dietary protein is required to attenuate muscle atrophy. There is preliminary, albeit somewhat speculative, evidence that specific interventions with supplementation of leucine or omega-3 fatty acids may attenuate the development of anabolic resistance and, as such, may help to retain muscle mass and function, thereby supporting subsequent rehabilitation.

Carbohydrate Ingestion

Carbohydrate intake during prolonged exercise increases endurance capacity and improves subsequent performance. Until recently, it was believed that carbohydrate intakes greater than 60–70 g per hour would not result in greater exogenous carbohydrate oxidation rates. In 'The New Carbohydrate Intake Recommendations', *Asker Jeukendrup* explains that recent work has revealed that exogenous carbohydrate oxidation rates can reach much higher values (up to 105 g/h) when multiple transportable carbohydrates are ingested (i.e. glucose and fructose). However, to allow absorption of such large amounts of carbohydrate, drinking needs to be trained. The gut has proven to be adaptable, and exogenous carbohydrate ingestion during exercise has to be trained by the competitive endurance athlete in preparing for competition. Obviously, all aspects of exercise competition need to be trained, including the nutritional practice that is required to maximize performance.

Protein Ingestion
Dietary protein ingestion after exercise stimulates muscle protein synthesis, inhibits protein breakdown and, as such, stimulates net muscle protein accretion following resistance as well as endurance type exercise. Protein ingestion during and/or immediately after exercise has been suggested to facilitate the skeletal muscle adaptive response to each exercise session, resulting in more effective muscle reconditioning. In 'Role of Dietary Protein in Post-Exercise Muscle Reconditioning', *Luc van Loon* underlines the important role of dietary protein to allow skeletal muscle tissue to adapt to the demands imposed upon by regular exercise training. A few basic guidelines are defined with regard to the preferred type and amount of dietary protein and the timing by which protein should be ingested. Ingestion of approximately 20 g (whey) protein during and/or immediately after each exercise session is sufficient for most athletes to maximize post-exercise muscle protein synthesis rates. A healthy diet with smart timing of the dietary protein ingestion after each bout of exercise will likely improve the skeletal muscle adaptive response to more prolonged exercise training and, as such, enhances training efficiency.

Immune Status
As injury is an unavoidable aspect of sports participation, sickness is also common for an athlete. In the chapter 'Nutritional Support to Maintain Proper Immune Status during Intense Training', *Michael Gleeson* explains that athletes engaging in intense exercise training may be at an increased risk of developing symptoms of minor respiratory illness. The latter causes an athlete to interrupt training, underperform or even to miss important competitions. The ingestion of ample dietary protein and sufficient micronutrients in the diet, intake of exogenous carbohydrate during exercise, and the use of probiotic or (plant) polyphenol-containing supplements are nutritional strategies that may help to maintain proper immune status during intense exercise training. However, it is important to note that nutrition is merely one of the many factors that modulate infection risk. There are many other strategies that can help to prevent the de-

velopment of immune function depression or reduce the degree of pathogen exposure and, as such, reduce infection risk. However, without a healthy diet it will be very difficult to maintain proper immune function during periods of increased physical stress.

β-Alanine

In the chapter 'Use of β-Alanine as an Ergogenic Aid', *Wim Derave* discusses the scientific basis for the use of β-alanine as an ergogenic aid. β-Alanine supplementation can be used as an effective nutritional strategy to augment performance capacity during high-intensity exercise activities. Similar to the discussions on the use of sodium bicarbonate and dietary nitrate, there are still numerous issues that need to be resolved regarding the modalities of β-alanine supplementation that optimize the ergogenic properties in the various types of exercise activities. Furthermore, work is warranted to assess whether more prolonged β-alanine supplementation can augment exercise training intensity and/or volume, thereby enhancing exercise training adaptation and efficiency.

Vitamin D

Dietary assessment studies have shown that many athletes do not meet the dietary intake recommendations for vitamin D. Vitamin D deficiency can compromise immune status and impair muscle function. There is much speculation on the need for vitamin D supplementation in athletes. In her chapter, *Enette Larson-Meyer* explains that a common reason for poor vitamin D status is lack of sufficient sun exposure, resulting in inadequate vitamin D synthesis. As a compromised vitamin D status can compromise an athlete's overall health and training efficiency, it is important to screen athletes routinely for vitamin D status and apply proper dietary interventions to achieve recommended vitamin D intake.

Weight Management

With obesity being more prevalent in the general population, more and more younger athletes come to their sport with the necessity to reduce bodyweight or improve body composition to allow peak performance. In the chapter 'Weight Management in the Performance Athlete', *Melinda Manore* explains to us that health professionals need to be prepared with effective and evidence-based dietary approaches to help the athlete achieve proper bodyweight targets while preparing for competition. To facilitate weight loss, retain muscle mass, and minimize the risk of developing eating disorders, athletes should be taught to consume a low-energy-dense diet allowing the consumption of a large volume of food while reducing energy intake. Furthermore, athletes should be stimulated to eat proper breakfasts, spread food and protein intake throughout the day, consume food after each exercise session, eliminate the excessive use of sweetened beverages, and avoid the use of popular weight loss diets.

Clinical Relevance

The aim of this workshop was to explore the properties of various nutritional interventions to modulate the adaptive response to exercise training and, as such, to identify dietary strategies that could increase exercise training efficiency. The various speakers have all provided a specific chapter in which they present the scientific evidence to suggest that we can modulate the complex interaction between nutrition and exercise through dietary cointervention. Scientific research in this area of interest is still quite limited, and new data are slowly emerging. We need to define targets for dietary intervention that can effectively modulate the adaptive response to prolonged exercise training. The latter is obviously of importance to the competitive athlete, but it has also important clinical relevance. In many preventative and therapeutic strategies, exercise has become accepted as a cornerstone in disease management. However, severely deconditioned people and more clinically compromised patient groups generally suffer from exercise intolerance, limiting the volume and intensity of the exercise that can be performed. In these conditions, a more efficient adaptive response to an increase in habitual physical activity and/or exercise training would likely translate to greater health benefits. Clearly, the relevance of nutritional coaching to modulate training efficiency will not be restricted to the competitive athlete, but also extends to the general public and more clinically compromised patient groups. There are many new challenges ahead to unravel the complex interaction between exercise and nutrition in both health and disease. More insight in this matter will help us to define effective nutritional strategies that can increase the benefits of regular exercise training to improve exercise performance and health.

Subject Index

Adaptation, *see* High-intensity interval training adaptation; Training adaptation
β-Alanine supplementation
    acidosis prevention and bicarbonate loading comparison 105–107
    bicarbonate loading combination 24, 25
    carnosine response in muscle 99–102
    dosing 25
    ergogenic mechanism 103, 104, 140
    exercise duration response 102, 103
    high-intensity interval training adaptation 46, 47
    history of study 100
    side effects 102
AMP-activated protein kinase (AMPK)
    exercise response 3
    glycogen availability effects on levels 4, 5
    high-intensity interval training adaptation 45

Beetroot juice, *see* Nitrate supplementation
Bicarbonate loading
    acidosis prevention and β-alanine supplementation comparison 105–107
    acute loading protocols 16, 17
    chronic use in training 21, 22
    high-intensity interval training adaptation 46, 49
    overview 15, 16, 137
    serial loading 18, 21
    side effects 25
    sports performance benefit studies 17–21
Bodyweight
    energy balance 125–127
    general population versus athletes 124, 125
    healthy bodyweight achieving 126–128, 141, 142
    weight loss diet
        breakfast 129–131
        fad diet avoidance 131
        high-calorie beverage avoidance 131
        low-energy-dense diet 128, 129
        meal timing 129–131
Bone
    immobilization response 57
    vitamin D function 112, 113

Caffeine, high-intensity interval training adaptation 49
Carbohydrate intake
    dose-response of exercise performance 66
    exercise duration recommendations 64–66, 71
    gut training and absorption capacity 66, 67, 139

immune depression prevention in
	intense training 89, 90
intermittent sports 67
mouth glucose 70, 71
post-exercise muscle
	reconditioning 78
practical limits 70
skill sports 67, 68
supplement forms 71
Carnosine, β-alanine effects in muscle
	99–102
Casein
muscle anabolism effects 61
post-exercise muscle
	reconditioning 77, 82
Chocolate, immunonutrition support for
	athletes 82
Colostrum, immunonutrition support for
	athletes 93
Creatine supplementation
β-alanine comparison 25
high-intensity interval training
	adaptation 49
Cytochrome oxidase (COX), high-
	intensity interval training
	adaptation 43

Dieting, see Bodyweight

Energy balance, factors regulating
	125–127

Fish oil, see Omega-6 fatty acids

GLUT4, immobilized muscle
	expression 55
Glycogen
high-intensity interval training
	adaptation 44
training adaptation
	endurance exercise recovery and
		substrate availability 7–10, 13,
		14
	muscle carbohydrate availability
		effects on cell metabolism
		acute effects 4–6
		chronic effects 6, 7, 136

Hexokinase II (HKII), exercise
	response 8
High-intensity interval training (HIT)
adaptation
	mechanisms 48, 49, 138
	metabolic factors limiting
		performance 42
	nutritional strategies 44–47, 49
	overview 42–44
	special populations 49

Immobilization, see Injury recovery
Immune status
immunonutrition support for athletes
	colostrum 93
	polyphenols 91, 92
	probiotics 92, 93, 96
infection types in athletes 96
intense training and depression
	nutrition strategies for prevention
		carbohydrate intake 89, 90
		endurance athletes 96
		practical recommendations 93,
			94, 139, 140
		supplements 87–89
		vitamin C 90, 91, 96, 97
	overview 85, 86
nutritional factors in maintenance 87,
	95, 96
Inflammation
injury recovery 52, 53
vitamin D anti-inflammatory
	activity 114
Injury recovery
bone, tendon, and ligament response
	to immobilization 57
energy intake recommendations 56,
	57, 60, 61
inflammatory response 52, 53
muscle response during immobility
	anabolic resistance 54, 55
	loss 53
	metabolism 55, 56
nutrition recommendations 57, 58,
	60, 138
nutritional status 52
vitamin D status in athletes 115

Leucine
  muscle loss prevention during
    immobilization 61
  muscle protein synthesis response 54,
    55
Ligament, response to immobilization 57
Lipoprotein lipase (LPL), exercise
  response 8

Maximal oxygen uptake, nitrate
  supplementation response 32–34
Mitochondrial P/O ratio, nitrate
  supplementation response 36

Nitrate supplementation
  exercise performance response 32–34
  mechanisms of action 34–36, 40
  nitric oxide pathway 27–29
  oxygen uptake response 29–32
  practical recommendations 36, 37, 40,
    137, 138
  side effects 39, 40
  vegetable content 28
Nitric oxide
  nitrate supplementation response, see
    Nitrate supplementation
Nuclear respiratory factor (NRF),
  mitochondria effects 3

Obesity, see Bodyweight
Omega-6 fatty acids, injury recovery
  anti-inflammatory action 53
  muscle loss prevention 55, 60
Oxygen uptake, nitrate supplementation
  response 29–32

Peroxisome proliferator-activated
  receptor-γ coactivator-1α (PGC-1α)
  exercise response 3–5
  high-intensity interval training
    adaptation 43
Phosphocreatine, nitrate supplementation
  response 35
Probiotics, immunonutrition support for
  athletes 92, 93, 96
Protein intake
  injury recovery 54

post-exercise muscle reconditioning
  amount of protein 75–77, 83
  carbohydrate effects 78
  endurance athletes 83
  practical recommendations 80, 139
  protein synthesis rates 74, 82
  rationale 75
  sources of protein 77, 78
  timing 78–80
pre-exercise effects 14
Pyruvate dehydrogenase kinase 4 (PDK4),
  exercise response 8

Quercetin, immunonutrition support for
  athletes 91, 92

Supplements, see β-Alanine
  supplementation; Casein; Creatine
  supplementation; Nitrate
  supplementation; Vitamin D

Tendon, response to immobilization 57
Training adaptation, see also High-
  intensity interval training adaptation
  endurance exercise recovery and
    substrate availability 7–10, 13, 14
  low-intensity training and training
    efficiency 10, 11, 14, 136
  muscle carbohydrate availability
    effects on cell metabolism
    acute effects 4–6
    chronic effects 6, 7, 136
  overview 1–4

Uncoupling protein 3 (UCP3), exercise
  response 8

Vitamin C, immune depression
  prevention in intense training 90, 91,
  96, 97
Vitamin D
  bone health during injury recovery 57
  deficiency and immune
    depression 87, 97
  functions
    anti-inflammatory activity 114
    bone 112, 113

immune response 113, 114
muscle 113
status in athletes
  assessment 117–119
  injury recovery 115
  overview 110–112
  performance effects 114, 115
  requirements 115, 116
supplementation 117, 119, 140
synthesis and sources 110, 111
toxicity 116

Weight, *see* Bodyweight
Whey, post-exercise muscle reconditioning 77, 82, 83